COURAGEOUS NEW DAWN

MASTERING YOUR MINDSET UNDERSTANDING ANXIETY - LEARNING TO THRIVE WITH FEAR IN AN EVER-CHANGING WORLD! - 2ND EDITION

WHAT TO DO FIRST SERIES

BOOK ONE

PETER A. LAST

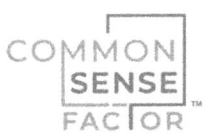

Published by CS Factor Book Publishing

Copyright – 1204843 © 2023 by Peter A. Last. All rights reserved.

No part of this publication may be reproduced, distributed, or transmitted in any form or by any means, including photocopying, recording, or other electronic or mechanical methods, without the prior written permission of the publisher, except in the case of brief quotations embodied in critical reviews and specific other non-commercial uses permitted by copyright law. For permission requests, write to the publisher, addressed:

Attention: Permissions Coordinator, at the address below.

CS Factor Book Publishing

admin@csfactor.com

Limit of Liability/Disclaimer of Warranty:

While the publisher and author have used their best efforts in preparing this book, they make no representations or warranties concerning the accuracy or completeness of the book's contents and specifically disclaim any implied warranties of merchantability or fitness for a particular purpose. Sales representatives or written sales materials may create or extend no warranty. Neither the publisher nor the author shall be liable for any loss of profit or other commercial damages, including but not limited to special, incidental, consequential, or other damages.

Courageous New Dawn – Mastering Your Mindset Understanding Anxiety - Learning to Thrive With Fear in an Ever-Changing World (2nd Edition) contains information on mindset growth and understanding fear and anxiety. The author has compiled this guide based on his own experiences and research. This information is not intended as medical advice, treatment plans, promises to overcome fear and anxiety, or an improved mindset – but rather an educational resource that may help you better understand the subject matter to make better choices for your journey.

Publishing and editorial team: CS Factor Book Publishing

Publishing Manager: P. Last

Editor: Abigail Gibbs

ISBN 978-1-7386889-7-5 E-Book

ISBN 978-1-7386889-8-2 Audio

ISBN 978-1-7381222-8-8 Paperback

ISBN 978-1-7381222-9-5 Hard Cover

Quantity Sales in paperback format are available. For details, contact the publisher at the email address above.

                        2nd Edition

Man Set Impressions

"Within the societal impressions set by man, especially during the Industrial Revolution, a culture emerged where suppressing emotions became a tool for increased productivity. It's time to break free from these constructed norms and embrace our true selves."

— COMMON SENSE FACTOR

This book is a dedication to the men and women of the world who have been molded by fear and anxiety, influencing who they are and how they interact with the world. It is a call to all men and women who may feel disconnected from their emotions and disconnected from their true desires. We have been programmed to follow a safe and steady path handed down to us from previous generations. We have been taught not to show emotion or vulnerability, which may reflect weakness. But at what cost?

Many of us have experienced childhood traumas that affect our confidence and ability to express ourselves fully. We hold in our feelings, not realizing that our emotions are essential to our being. We must allow ourselves to feel, to express ourselves, and to embrace our true desires. It takes strength to acknowledge our fears and vulnerabilities and courage to confront them.

It's time to break the cycle of non-emotional responses and limitations ingrained in us for generations. We must let go of the fear of being judged as weak or vulnerable and understand that it is okay to show emotion. By confronting our anxieties and traumas, we can begin to heal and live a life filled with joy, purpose, and connection.

So, to all the men and women, understand that your fear and anxiety do not define you. It's time to be direct and firm as we confront our emotions and embrace our true selves. Let us break free from the limiting belief system and strive for a life filled with happiness and fulfillment.

When I am afraid, I put my trust in you.

— PSALM 56:3

FOREWORD

As I reflect back on the time I have known Peter, what truly stands out is his commitment to helping others cultivate a courageous mindset. As our world continues to evolve and change, this capacity for courage may very well be the key to unlocking our fullest potential. His book not only provides valuable insights into how we can develop our own courage but also encourages us to become inspired to find our own path.

Peter's **B. B.R.A.V.E** framework serves as a roadmap for moving through our fears and anxieties to reach our fullest potential and be more courageous in life. It is divided into six distinct categories, all of which are essential pieces of the puzzle when it comes to personal growth: **B** – Banishing Fear, **B** – Breaking Negative Patterns, **R** – Revising Core Beliefs, **A** – Adopting Mindfulness, **V** – Vanquishing Procrastination and **E** – Embracing Growth and Thriving. Each of these areas is examined in detail throughout the book and provides practical tools and strategies for working through them.

The 'Courageous New Dawn' offers a unique opportunity to gain insight into Peter's perspective on the power of courage and how it can be used to navigate our lives. It also serves as a reminder that we all have the capacity for courageousness, and with the right mindset, anything is possible. It's an absolute honor to be asked to write this foreword, and I hope it will help readers find their courage and reach new heights of success!

 Creator of The Implicit Career Search, Career Hero, and Working on Purpose

— STEVE MILLER

PREFACE

"The B Brave Framework"

In the heart of the night, when silence does yawn,
Rises a strength, the "Courageous New Dawn".
With every challenge every curve life may throw,
There's a framework we follow, a path we must know.
Begin with belief in your heart and your soul,
Believe in your power; let this be your goal.
For bravery starts where doubts fade away,
With every new challenge, you'll keep fear at bay.
Brave every storm with resolve and with might,
For darkness is fleeting, soon there'll be light.
The struggles you face, the pain that you bear,
Are stepping stones to greatness, a chance to prepare.

Rise from the ashes, like a phoenix so free,
With wings spread wide open, over land, over sea.
Every setback you've faced, every tear that you've shed,
Will fuel your ascent to the skies up ahead.
Awaken your spirit, let your inner child play,
Find joy in the moments; let it light up your day.
For the laughter of youth, the dreams so profound,
Will bring back the magic in life that's unbound.
Venture forth boldly, with courage and grace,
Every mountain, every challenge, you're ready to face.
With hope in your heart and fire in your eyes,
You'll conquer your fears and seize the prize.
Endure, for the journey, it's long, and it's tough,
But with the B. Brave framework, you're more than enough.
For at the end of the journey, with the battles you've strived,
With "Courageous New Dawn," you'll surely thrive.
So, embrace this new dawn with the B. Brave guide,
Together, we rise with courage and pride.
For the future's bright, with dreams to be drawn,
In the light of hope, with the "Courageous New Dawn".

— PETER A LAST

CONTENTS

Introduction	15
About the Author	23

1. UNDERSTANDING THE PSYCHOLOGICAL
   IMPACT OF THE PANDEMIC — 27
   - What is Human Vibration? — 29
   - Most Common Psychological Reactions to the COVID-19 Infection — 43
   - State of the Post-Pandemic World — 45
   - Relatable Stories — 49
   - Navigating the New Normal: Adapting to Change — 50
   - Challenges of Adapting to the New Normal and What to Do — 53
   - The Importance of Mindset — 58
   - The B. B.R.A.V.E. Framework — 61

2. BANISHING FEAR, WORRY, AND ANXIETY
   WITH A NEW PERSPECTIVE — 63
   - What Is Codependency? — 67
   - How to Overcome Fear and Anxiety — 75
   - Techniques to Treat Anxiety — 77
   - Tips to Overcome Fear and Anxiety — 80
   - Embracing and Harnessing Anxiety for Growth and Resilience — 84
   - Ways to Use Anxiety as a Source for Growth — 86
   - Develop Optimism and Mental Resilience to Conquer Anxiety — 92
   - Use These Tips to Increase Your Mental Resilience — 93
   - Relatable Stories — 99

3. BREAKING NEGATIVE THOUGHT PATTERNS — 101
   - Definition of Negative Thoughts or Hungry Ghosts — 104
   - Types of Negative Thoughts — 106

Increased Risk of Obsessive-Compulsive Disorder
(OCD)   111
Actionable Ways to Turn Negative Thinking into
Positive Thinking   114
Relatable Stories   114
Shifting Perspectives on Fear, Worry, and Anxiety   115

4. REVISING CORE BELIEFS   121
Where Do Core Beliefs Come From?   126
Core Beliefs: How They Influence You and What
to Do About It   127
Relatable Stories   131
Restructuring and Adopting Empowering Core
Beliefs   133
Reframing Defeating Beliefs and Language   143

5. ADOPTING MINDFULNESS   147
Mindfulness Exercises   154
Cultivating Present-Moment Awareness   156
How to Cultivate Present-Moment Awareness   161
Relatable Stories   164

6. VANQUISHING PROCRASTINATION   167
Understanding the Psychology of Procrastination   169
Building Motivation and Discipline to Take
Action   176
Relatable Stories   181

7. EMBRACING SUSTAINABLE GROWTH AND
THRIVING   183
Consistency and Habits   184
Growth and Learning   187
Relatable Stories   193

8. CELEBRATING YOUR JOURNEY OF
PERSONAL TRANSFORMATION   195
Embracing Gratitude and Joy   196
Setting New Goals and Continued Growth   204
What Are the Benefits of Goal Setting?   207
Reward Yourself   215

Relatable Stories 215
Interactive Elements 216

Conclusion 227
References 231

INTRODUCTION

 Fear and Anxiety are soul messages to be listened to!

— COMMON SENSE FACTOR

Three years ago, we faced one of the biggest global crises in generations. The COVID-19 pandemic had us all locked up in our own homes, economies collapsed, lives were lost, relationships strained and damaged, and many people were left with despair and uncertainty. The effects are not a laughing matter; for many years, we've tried to address the importance of mental well-being, and today, it has become more of a pressing issue. We might agree that the virus is no longer a threat, but what are the consequences of this tragedy?

Mental health is something that we need to pay attention to. However, not many people realize this. Throughout history, mental health has been perceived as something invisible—an invalid realm in our psyche. The fight to take mental health into value has been going on for centuries, and today, we need to address the importance of mental health even more.

The challenges of the pandemic may have faded for some, but for many, the repercussions are here to stay. Now, more than ever, harnessing the strength of our mindset is paramount. It's time for us to prioritize mental health, not as a passing concern but as a core aspect of our overall well-being and survival.

This book will delve deep into how our mindset can influence our overall health and success. Imagine navigating the post-pandemic world, not with dread, but with a clarity of purpose and optimism. The idea of a growth mindset isn't just theoretical. During the pandemic, Jim Carrey demonstrated a growth mindset by embracing new hobbies, such as painting and sharing his work on social media. He also encouraged his followers to stay positive and enjoy the small things.

As you turn these pages, understand that our shared wisdom will guide us. The essence is simple: to grow together, to support, and most importantly, to refrain from passing judgment on our peers. Dive in, and let's embark on this growth, resilience, and understanding journey together.

In these pages, you will also learn how to:

- **Take actionable steps:** You will be encouraged to take action for your well-being through interactive elements, allowing you to manage anxiety and fear better in the future.
- **Adopt science-backed strategies:** By providing you with methods and strategies proven by scientific research, I believe you can effectively make any desired healthy changes.
- **Practice personalized plans:** This book is tailored to guide you to develop healthy habits through personalized plans.
- **Learn about real-life experiences, case studies, and stories:** real-life examples will allow you to learn from others, making this book feel especially relatable.
- **Practice self-assessment tools:** tools and techniques for self-assessment will be provided to help you quickly identify triggers and stressors so you can better understand your anxiety patterns.
- Understanding the **complexities** of that protected inner child, the defense mechanisms you may have set in your early years, and how to set him/her free to overcome fear and anxiety.

Learning is a process; we encourage self-growth. It may take some time, but I assure you, the journey is worth it. The knowledge from this book can be read and digested in less than a week if you put your mind to it.

BENEFITS AND OUTCOMES OF READING THIS BOOK

After reading this book, you will have a more comprehensive idea about the importance of nurturing mental health and incorporating a growth mindset.

In this book, you will:

- Develop an understanding of your anxiety and fear, why you might experience these responses and feelings, and the mechanisms of anxiety and fear, especially after facing this global pandemic.
- Understand your inner child's healing needs, which may cause many of your fears and anxieties that have been buried by emotional suppression or repression. You'll understand and break barriers in your defense mechanisms and why you have placed them there.
- Understand what emotions can and will affect your vibration and why.
- Learn about codependency, how it affects you, and its deafening effect on fear and anxiety.
- Learn about the collective consciousness, the difference between it and group consciousness, and how it affects fear and anxiety.
- You will receive practical, holistic, scientifically-backed strategies to help you cope more effectively with stress and uncertainty.
- Learn how to manage negative emotions and improve your emotional well-being, leading to a happier life.
- Find practical guidance for life after the pandemic,

insights, and essential knowledge to help you navigate the changes in this post-pandemic world.

Now, visualize a life in which fear and anxiety are no longer prevalent. Instead of dreading the hurdles that await you in the morning, you approach it with a bright smile, an open heart, and an open mind. Anxiety, which was once a persistent shadow in the back of your mind, has now been replaced by confidence, tranquility, and peace. It hasn't gone away totally; it still exists on the outer edges of your mind, but you have more understanding of it now, and a constant flow of negative thoughts and feelings no longer chains you.

You're focused on the task at work, unaffected by the amount of work or stress that would normally set your mind spinning. You've discovered how to deal with disasters with elegance and comfort. Your relationships with others have deepened because you are no longer disturbed by the anxieties and fears that previously affected your thoughts and behaviors. The people closest to you will notice a positive change in how you act and respect you as a new person.

You are no longer concerned about what tomorrow may bring. Instead, you will concentrate on expressing gratitude for what you have experienced today: all of life's simple joys and small acts of kindness. You'll fall asleep quickly at night and wake up ready to face the next day.

You've learned how to regulate your emotions effectively, preparing yourself to succeed in a world changed by the pandemic. You will face the new normal with increased resilience that has been hardened while remaining adaptable to future problems.

You're not just surviving in this post-pandemic world but thriving confidently. No matter what challenges come your way, you'll face them bravely using the knowledge and skills you've gained. This is the revolutionary effect of a *Courageous New Dawn*: your dream life is becoming a reality.

I aim to make "common sense" effective for developing strong and healthy relationships. I have researched top experts in the fields of mindset, fear, and anxiety to find the most up-to-date knowledge on these subjects, which, combined with an in-depth knowledge of human behavior and communication, I believe will help you on your healing journey. My advice is theoretical and practical to encourage lasting positive change in your life.

I have dealt with anxiety disorders from an early age, not truly being aware of its control over my life until the pandemic made things much worse. However, by mastering my thinking and being present with myself, I've saved myself from these struggles and managed them effectively.

I believe in the power of empathy, compassion, and patience to help others adopt an optimistic mindset. I've seen how devastating unresolved thoughts can be, which motivates me to assist others in finding peaceful endings to their worries and anxieties. I believe in the power of shared knowledge and the lasting impacts it can leave for significant change. This book will be a beacon of light to guide you through conquering your mindset and beginning a more mindful, peaceful life from now on.

Join me in this opportunity to master your mindset. Let's work together to make sense of the chaos, keeping the Common Sense Factor in mind.

> "You must determine where you are going in your life, because you cannot get there unless you move in that direction. Random wandering will not move you forward. It will instead disappoint and frustrate you and make you anxious and unhappy and hard to get along with (and then resentful, and then vengeful, and then worse)."
>
> — DR. JORDAN B. PETERSON

If you get inspired while reading and would like to join a group of like-minded individuals on Facebook
HEALTHY BODY - HEALTHY MIND
at CommonSenseFactor.us

ABOUT THE AUTHOR

Have you ever felt the world's weight on your shoulders, the pain that shapes your life? Imagine being Peter Last, who, from the young age of 7, bore the emotional scars of his parents' divorce. This early trauma, a silent companion that followed him, manifested as anxiety and later evolved into codependency traits, shaping much of his adult life. But Peter wasn't one to simply accept this. Much like you might seek answers in challenging times, he embarked on a transformative journey to find possible healing methods.

In 2014, eager for tools and techniques to navigate his inner landscape, Peter trained as a hypnotist. Picture the power of diving deep into the subconscious, unlocking past traumas, and reframing them. That's the potential he harnessed. Recognizing the intimate connection between mind and body, he further honed his skills as a health coach in 2015.

Think back to the onset of the pandemic, a time when uncertainty hovered in the air. For Peter, the lockdowns amplified his familiar anxious feelings. Yet, he channeled this into creativity, penning "Got Smoothie Go – It's A Nutrient Rich Life – Your Smoothie Guide to Detox, Fighting Disease, Muscle Health,

Healthy Weight Loss & Vibrant Living." It became more than a book; it marked the start of his publishing venture, Common Sense Factor Book Publishing. Can you feel his drive? His mission is clear: to sprinkle practical wisdom into everyday lives, much like he sought for himself.

Over the past three years, as you've perhaps navigated your own challenges, Peter faced his anxiety anew. This self-examination birthed another masterpiece, "Courageous New Dawn: Mastering Your Mindset Understanding Anxiety - Learning to Thrive with Fear in an Ever-Changing World!" As you delve into his words, Peter wants you to grasp one crucial message: you are never alone in your battles. Whether you're grappling with anxiety, fear, or any other challenge, there's hope, healing, and an astounding strength within you. Every day, as Peter confronts his hurdles, he's committed to lighting the way for others, guiding them to a sanctuary of well-being and a heart full of empathy.

Head into these pages with an open heart and mind, and you might find echoes of your journey and the inspiration to forge ahead.

C - Compassionate
O - Optimistic
M - Mindful
M - Motivated
O - Observant
N - Nurturing

S - Sincere
E - Empathetic
N - Nonjudgmental
S - Self-aware
E - Ethical

F - Forward-thinking
A - Adaptable
C - Cognizant
T - Tolerant
O - Objective
R - Resilient

Visit The Author's Page @
AuthorEnd.com

1

UNDERSTANDING THE PSYCHOLOGICAL IMPACT OF THE PANDEMIC

> *When the physical threat of coronavirus subsides, as it surely will, we must address the impact on our mental health.*
>
> — LUCIANA BERGER

As a new chapter unfolds after the pandemic, there's a beacon of hope and a chance for fresh beginnings. Yet, amid the swell of optimism, you might feel an undercurrent of anxiety, sensing the immense global shifts still unfolding and evolving. As you venture into this unfamiliar landscape of the post-pandemic world, it's crucial for you to acknowledge the realities facing you and to equip yourself with the transformative B-BRAVE framework, which will be detailed later on. You stand at the threshold of a journey toward self-discovery, resilience, and mental well-being in a world undergoing irrevocable change.

Even if the physical signs aren't always evident, studies reveal that the pandemic's feelings of isolation, stress, fear, and frustration have deeply affected many people's mental well-being. The ramifications of the pandemic aren't just about the virus; they pierce deep into the realm of psychological health. As you grapple with these invisible challenges, focusing on and prioritizing mental health becomes paramount, as is finding paths through this emotional labyrinth to rediscover balance amidst the chaos.

Through your exploration and understanding of the latest research, it's evident that mental well-being has suffered considerably in recent years. You might come across studies like the one by Serra and colleagues (2022) that spotlighted the prevalence of PTSD among COVID-19 patients. Discovering that about 11% of these individuals grapple with chronic PTSD is a wake-up call, especially with rising anxiety disorders, depression, and other mental health conditions.

Has the storm of the pandemic indeed passed? Can you return to what once felt like **"normal"**? Consider this: humanity has faced one of the gravest global crises since World War II. Reflecting on the stories of those like your grandfather—a man deeply scarred by the horrors of war, whose anger and pain seemed trapped in time—might make you wonder if society is at a pivotal juncture that has forever shifted the communal trajectory.

In this chapter, you'll dive deep into the enduring mental health aftermath of the pandemic. You'll grasp the significance of safeguarding your mental equilibrium in the face of global disasters, chronic ailments, distrust, frustration, and feelings of isolation.

This exploration will encompass the myriad ways people react to hardships. You're about to embark on an enlightening journey through the multifaceted realm of post-crisis mental health, underscoring the essence of self-love, self-compassion and empathy towards others as you chart these waters.

WHAT IS HUMAN VIBRATION?

Human vibration is the concept that every individual emits a specific frequency or energy pattern. This frequency is influenced by one's emotions, thoughts, physical health, and overall well-being. Positive emotions like love and joy tend to raise one's vibrational frequency, while negative emotions like anger and fear can lower it. Some believe we can align more closely with our authentic selves and the universe by understanding and tuning into our vibrations, leading to enhanced spiritual, emotional, and physical health.

Examining the Long-Term Effects of the Pandemic on Mental Health

By deeply exploring the pandemic's lasting impacts, you'll understand the vital role of mental resilience. Recognizing how the pandemic has touched your psyche and what might be on the horizon is crucial, preparing you to face future challenges with grace and strength.

Navigating the numerous mental health hurdles after the pandemic, it's also essential for you to understand the evolving world around you and find your footing amidst these changes.

It's natural to feel a sense of unease considering the magnitude of transformations and the realization that some things may never revert to what they once were. But here's where your mental resilience shines: empowering you to embrace and thrive amidst these shifts. Moreover, cultivating mindfulness by shifting your perspective and mindset will be a beacon of light in these times. This chapter guides you through resilience and mindfulness, supporting you at every step.

By fostering a nurturing and inclusive approach to addressing mental health issues, you are setting the stage for your healing and contributing to a brighter, more compassionate future for people everywhere.

How COVID-19 Has Affected Mental Health

Perception of truth becomes a reality, constantly questioning the information provided.

— COMMON SENSE FACTOR

How exactly did the pandemic influence your mental well-being? The key isn't solely in your perception of the virus but also in how society responded to it.

You might have felt the pandemic like a whirlwind of emotions. Initially, you could've been swamped by the relentless influx of information about the virus's dangers, its health consequences, and the alarming death rates. Perhaps you were left pondering numerous questions, especially when some of the symptoms of the virus, like fatigue, mirrored your physical feelings after a long day of construction work. *Could I have been exposed to the virus without knowing?* you might've wondered. The origins, causes, and details about the virus became a swirl of information and misinformation. Soon, various narratives, including conspiracy theories, clouded the waters, making it hard to differentiate genuine information from mere speculation.

The rapid societal shifts due to the pandemic, combined with the profound reactions of so many, undoubtedly weighed heavily on your heart. Remember, feeling this way is natural; you're not alone in navigating these complex emotions. With grim news dominating the headlines and instances of violence, racism, and intolerance rising, it could've felt like the world was turning darker. Yet, amidst this chaos, remember the love, compassion, and unity many shared. Remember that in the face of adversity, our **collective strength** and kindness have the power to heal.

Here are a few main reasons why the pandemic had such a significant effect on our psychological health.

Interconnected Emotions: Navigating Collective and Group Consciousness in Challenging Times

When you think about collective consciousness, a concept introduced by sociologist Émile Durkheim, you're diving into the shared beliefs, values, attitudes, and knowledge that a community or society holds. Consider the global response to COVID-19: it's as if we, together as a worldwide family, experienced a shared emotional and mental journey. But then there are moments, like the Freedom Convoy, that serve as a testament to group consciousness. When a specific group, driven by shared identities or experiences—like concerns over vaccine mandates or individual rights—comes into the spotlight. This consciousness is more focused, representing a subgroup within the broader society.

Understanding these dynamics is vital, especially when considering their impact on well-being. If you're in a society where the majority feel anxious due to various factors, you might still feel that shared sense of unease even if you're not directly affected. It's a testament to our interconnectedness, we are one. On the other hand, if you belong to a group facing challenges, that group consciousness can affect your peace of mind, especially if you feel marginalized or threatened. Remember, it's natural to feel these collective emotions, and recognizing their origins is the first step towards navigating them with grace and compassion.

"In this scenario, I've learned that feeling and understanding rational and irrational thoughts need to be addressed, we'll cover these thought patterns later in the book. Understand that behind each action, from anyone, group or government underlies a specific outcome. First, does it benefit you; second does it affect you or your family and third is it vital to mankind."

How Social Media Affects: Collective and Group Consciousness in Challenging Times

When you scroll through your social media feeds, you're not just glimpsing the lives of friends and celebrities. You're tapping into a modern manifestation of collective consciousness. Platforms like Facebook, Twitter, and Instagram can magnify shared emotions, beliefs, and experiences across global communities. During challenging times, such as a worldwide pandemic or significant social movements, you might notice these platforms brimming with synchronized sentiments, echoing the collective mood of society.

Imagine a ripple in a pond; one influential post or viral trend can send waves across the digital realm, influencing how you and countless others perceive and react to events. Especially true for group consciousness. For instance, a hashtag can spotlight a specific group's struggles or triumphs, bringing attention to shared identities or experiences that might have previously been overlooked. As you engage with these digital movements, you may feel a heightened sense of connection, solidarity, or even conflict with others.

However, with the power of social media also comes its challenges. The echo chambers, the potential for misinformation, and the speed at which emotions can escalate can sometimes be overwhelming. If ever you find the weight of collective emotions heavy on your heart or feel swayed by the intense hunger of group consciousness, remember *"If it bleeds, it leads" A cross-national study suggests consumers around the world have stronger psychophysiological reactions to negative news when compared to positive news. The report is one of the largest of its kind and was published in (2019)* PNAS. *Always, remember* to step back and breathe.

It's okay to disconnect, reflect, and seek authentic offline connections. After all, while social media offers a window into collective moods, proper understanding and compassion come from nurturing personal relationships and introspection. Remember, it's a tool for connection, but your well-being and understanding always come first.

*"**These tools** will feed your fear and anxiety; they've fed mine, access everything with critical thinking practices; we'll discuss these a little further in the book."*

False Rumors and News

Navigating through the pandemic wasn't just about facing the disease; it was also about wading through the overwhelming reactions and emotions of those around you. Misinformation on safety measures, rampant rumors, and an ever-churning news cycle could have distorted your view of others. The omnipresent media might have intensified your fears, especially on social media platforms. Even amidst words of reassurance, it became increasingly challenging for you to know whom to trust. While vaccines have been developed and healthcare systems have improved, uncertainties linger—stories of legal cases, profits, and patents associated with the vaccine technology have emerged (ncbi.nlm.nih.gov). But genuinely understanding or untangling these tales would take more than discerning eyes. Remember, sometimes, letting go and focusing on elevating your well-being is the most compassionate act you can offer to yourself and the world as a whole.

"Now that we've discussed collective and group consciousness, the news can be presented in such a way to ultimately lower the vibration of humanity, so negative news is an energy vampire, lowering your vibration and allowing limiting beliefs (hungry ghosts) in, protect your energy."

"While running my renovation business during the pandemic, I came across conflicting information; the local health unit was mandating mask-wearing, so I reviewed the guidelines to ensure that myself and staff were complying safely. Yet, one of the mentions on the health website was that a mask may be temporarily taken off **"if to engage in an athletic or fitness activity."**

Well, for those who have experienced construction work, it's a physical job, perspiration happening, masks absorb the perspiration, making it harder to breathe, the potential for oxygen deprivation, passing out, falling, impaling yourself on a sharp object around the site. This escalated to the Occupational Health and Safety Board, then up to the Human Rights Board. Can you feel my anxiety and stress levels rising!"

Disruption to Mental Health Services

You and many others found yourselves in a world where healthcare workers were tirelessly battling COVID-19, making it challenging to prioritize comprehensive mental health services. Can you imagine? A 2020 survey by the World Health Organization revealed that 93% of mental health services faced disruptions or complete shutdowns due to the pandemic. The need came when you and many others sought mental health support more than ever. Heartbreakingly, even before the pandemic, most nations allocated less than 2% of their budgets to mental healthcare. These resources were directed towards general hospitals that were already stretched thin, trying to cater to the physical health needs of their citizens. They underscored how the mental well-being of individuals like you may have felt overlooked or undervalued for far too long. Remember, your mental health matters, and you must continue advocating for the support you deserve.

"In my generational era, for me to openly admit that I had mental challenges, the ridicule I would have received would have sent me over the top; I had already set defense mechanisms that were very comfortable at the time. More on Inner Child Trauma a little later in the book."

Social Isolation

During the pandemic, you, like so many others, endured the effects of lockdowns, social distancing, and stringent safety measures worldwide. Public spaces became off-limits, and the gentle encouragement to stay home became a heavy weight of isolation. This lack of human connection, fundamental to our essence, likely weighed on your heart, according to a survey by Queen's University Belfast reported by ScienceDaily in 2020, over 26.6% of individuals admitted to feeling an intensified sense of loneliness. Being away from friends, family, and dear ones wasn't just a physical distance but an emotional chasm. Remember, it's natural to feel this way, especially when we understand loneliness can be closely tied to other emotional challenges, like depression. Know that in these feelings, there's strength and healing in recognizing and sharing them.

"Don't feed down, feed up, write or read a book, try something new that excites you, be creative, it's in you!"

Weakened Economy and Financial Burdens

You've undoubtedly felt the ripple effects of this global health crisis as so many countries have been striving to cope. Over recent years, the world you once knew changed, witnessing a dip in economic activity that likely touched you or those close to you. Jobs were lost, cherished businesses closed, and sectors like tourism, retail, and hospitality, which many depended on, came to a standstill.

When 2020 rolled along, the world you traversed became more restricted, with lockdowns and curtailed global mobility. It's heart-wrenching to think that around 114 million individuals, possibly friends, family, or even yourself, were nudged into unemployment. These impacts weren't just numbers or headlines; they resonated deeply, influencing personal finances, taking away community hubs, and altering life as you knew it.

And through this, it's entirely understandable if your mental well-being felt strained. The weight of this economic setback surpassed even 2008-2009, coined The Great Recession, stripping away an estimated $3.7 trillion in earnings. It's essential to remember that in these feelings or experiences. These trying times call for love, patience, and understanding for ourselves and those around us (Richter, 2021).

New Mental Health Conditions vs. Existing Mental Illnesses: How COVID-19 Impacted Both

The pandemic undeniably presented immense challenges, especially for those of you already navigating mental health battles and those who had been untouched by them. The unfortunate reduction in mental health resources, rising societal complexities, and the world's unsettling state left many searching for ways to cope. Some of you might have felt the pull towards smoking, increased alcohol intake, drug use, or other forms of substance reliance as a way to escape the pressure momentarily.

From December 2020, the statistics showed a concerning uptick in drug-related fatalities and thoughts of self-harm. The Centers for Disease Control and Prevention (C.D.C.) highlighted that an alarming 13% of U.S. citizens found themselves leaning on potentially harmful substances to navigate the challenges of the pandemic (Czeisler, 2020).

"Please remember, you're never alone in this journey. Understanding these realities, allowing them, acknowledging them, and seeking healthier coping methods is the first step toward healing. Your strength and resilience are commendable, and the community here is ready to support and embrace you with love and compassion."

The Effects of Long COVID on Mental Health

Long COVID describes the symptoms you might experience for weeks or even months after recovering from the immediate phase of a COVID-19 infection. Please know the impact of Long COVID on your mental well-being can be diverse and profound. Remember, it's okay to seek support and understanding as you navigate these challenges.

- **Chronic Fatigue:** You may be experiencing persistent fatigue, a common symptom of Long COVID. This constant tiredness can make daily tasks feel overwhelming and might even amplify feelings of depression or anxiety.
- **Cognitive Difficulties:** You might sometimes feel what many affectionately call brain fog, where focusing, recalling memories, or processing thoughts becomes challenging. Experiencing this can understandably lead to frustration and strain in your personal and professional life.
- **Mood Disorders:** Long COVID might cause you to experience shifts in your mood, potentially leading to challenges like anxiety and depression. These feelings could arise as a response to the ongoing physical discomfort or the virus's direct biological effect on your body.
- **PTSD and Trauma-Related Disorders:** For those of you who endured severe bouts of COVID-19 and found yourselves needing hospital care, the harrowing

experience of the illness might have left deep imprints on your psyche. It's understandable if such experiences have given rise to feelings akin to post-traumatic stress disorder (PTSD) or other emotional challenges.

- **Sleep Disturbances:** Shifts in your sleep patterns or bouts of insomnia might be linked to Long COVID. When you're deprived of restful sleep, it can deeply touch every facet of your mental well-being. It can influence your mood, cloud your thinking, and affect your overall wellness.
- **Social Isolation:** The lasting impacts of Long COVID might limit your ability to participate in social gatherings, possibly causing you to feel isolated and lonely. These feelings can be linked to various mental health struggles.
- **Existential Stress:** Long COVID-19's ongoing uncertainty might make you feel deeply anxious about your future health and well-being. Please know that such feelings are valid, and grappling with such concerns is natural during these challenging times.

Recognizing the mental health implications of Long COVID is vital for you and the broader community. It's essential to understand that the effects of COVID-19 aren't just about the immediate phase of the infection. You might find that it has prolonged and varied impacts on your mental well-being.

It's not only about healing physically but also about understanding and navigating the emotional and mental hurdles that Long COVID may present. In the face of these new symptoms evolving, you're facing new challenges and deserve compassion and support every step of the way.

Why Good Mental Health is Important for Chronic Illness Sufferers

 To keep the body in good health is a duty... otherwise, we shall not be able to keep our minds strong and clear.

— BUDDHA

Your physical and mental well-being are deeply intertwined. If you're battling chronic conditions like diabetes, cancer, or heart disease, understand that these might also impact your mental health. Conversely, if your mental well-being is compromised, it can manifest in physical ailments over time. It's genuinely said that a troubled mind can lead to a troubled body. Research suggests that those grappling with depression may have a higher risk of stroke, Alzheimer's disease, and diabetes, especially if they find solace in food.

Facing a chronic condition is challenging, and with the added stress of the pandemic, it becomes even more taxing. Know that your mental well-being is a beacon of strength. Nurturing a positive mindset uplifts your spirit and empowers you to navigate daily challenges with grace and resilience. Remember, you deserve love, understanding, and support in all facets of your journey.

The Psychological Impact of Being in Quarantine

As the world changed around you, the impact of government-imposed lockdown policies was felt deeply. You were classified as an essential worker, and while your work schedule persisted or even intensified, you couldn't help but empathize with those parents who once took pride in supporting their families and were now labeled as non-essential. A challenging mental hurdle to surpass, indeed.

Suddenly, familiar faces at school became distant memories, and the long-awaited visits to cherished family members were halted. Imagine longing to see a beloved aunt in her final moments, only to be told that visitations were restricted; *I'm* speaking from *the* heart here. The weight of the lockdown wasn't just physical but profoundly mental; while being bound within the walls of your home, gatherings became a thing of the past, and even deeply personal events like funerals were curtailed, all hoping to halt the virus's spread.

This sudden shift birthed feelings of isolation and loneliness, sapping the joy from daily life and putting a strain on your mental well-being. As days turned into weeks, trust in governmental and health authorities started to waver. The very bonds that connected you with family and friends felt like they were fraying; they had broken down silently, **adding another layer to emotional challenges.**

MOST COMMON PSYCHOLOGICAL REACTIONS TO THE COVID-19 INFECTION

As you became more informed about the spread of the COVID-19 infection, your emotional response might have ranged from concern to overwhelming anxiety. You might have noticed people around you beginning to stock up on supplies, sometimes not considering the needs of others and, in extreme cases, even resorting to aggression to secure what they felt was essential. Looking back, these actions appear excessive, but most of us hadn't faced such uncertainties before, and survival instincts kicked in. Your apprehensions about the future amidst all this chaos were completely valid. In its unrelenting wake, the pandemic likely revealed both challenging and inspiring facets of our collective humanity.

Here are some reflections on the prevalent psychological responses to the spread of the COVID-19 infection during those trying times:

Specific and Uncontrolled Fears Related to Infection

You might have often found yourself deeply concerned about your health, haunted by the idea of passing the virus to someone else or catching it yourself. It's understandable, especially when conflicting information about COVID-19 spread across different regions or communities, causing confusion and apprehension. Even minor symptoms like a sore throat, fever, or sneeze might have made you wonder if you were contagious, amplifying your worries. Research suggests that these concerns might have been even more pronounced if you were pregnant or lived with young children. It's as if your natural defense mechanism was trying to protect you but was driven by fear. Remember, feeling this way is okay; you're not alone in your concerns.

Pervasive Anxiety

When faced with social isolation and lockdown measures, you might have felt a surge of anxiety, a natural response when confronted with the unfamiliar. There was so much unknown about this virus, yet its rapid spread was undeniable. Concerns about the future were hard to shake, especially with the emergence of mutating variants like the COVID Delta or the COVID Omicron. Please know that such feelings were shared by many, and it's completely understandable to have felt this way. *We're in this together,* as mentioned in many newscasts.

"In the face of uncertainty and isolation, remember that our shared emotions are a testament to our collective strength. Together, we navigate the unknown and emerge resilient."

Frustration and Boredom

A lack of physical touch and deep connections with others led to feelings of frustration and monotony. You've felt it too, haven't you? Those simple joys, like meeting a friend for a mid-week chat and a drink, were suddenly off the table. Your days probably seemed endless, almost reaching a breaking point, showcasing just how influential our mindsets can be. Being apart from those you care about might have sapped your motivation for daily routines. Perhaps you couldn't go to work or faced job loss, upending the rhythm of your daily life. Some might have even felt trapped within their own homes. With outside activities off limits and the struggle to combat boredom, you might have encountered deep-seated feelings of despair, isolation, and loneliness. Remember, you're not alone in this journey; seeking support and understanding is okay.

"A neighbor once shared her feelings of restlessness with me, watching me leave for work every day. She wondered where I was headed. While her job was considered non-essential, she was thankful to have the option of working from home. Still, her conversation revealed a deep desire for social interaction."

STATE OF THE POST-PANDEMIC WORLD

The world around you has transformed in the wake of the pandemic, especially in areas like technological advancement and the suggested blossoming digital economy. Perhaps you've felt a shift towards preferring non-physical contact for daily tasks. These evolving trends surround you, touching various facets of life. Maybe you've found solace in remote work or learning, adapted to new modes of communication, or felt the pinch of inflation. With the surge in online health services and shifts in the labor market, it's clear the post-pandemic world has reshaped the environment in ways that resonate deeply with you. Remember, it's okay to take a moment to adjust and find your footing in this ever-changing landscape.

People Who Struggled Before Now Struggle More

If you've faced financial hardships, grappled with existing mental or physical health issues, or belong to racialized and marginalized communities, these times might feel especially daunting for you. The pandemic and post-pandemic struggles, economic downturns, and rising inflation might have intensified your challenges. If you were already navigating financial constraints, securing basic necessities like food might feel even more overwhelming now.

As the pandemic unfolded, I watched in concern as supply chain disruptions escalated and the cost of essential items surged. What used to cost me forty to fifty dollars every few days has now shockingly doubled. Experiencing these changes firsthand, I can't help but wonder: Given the global magnitude of this pandemic, why weren't measures put in place, similar to the Nixon Shock in 1971, that addressed inflation? (Wikipedia) It feels like the signs were there, yet someone has dropped the ball on this important preventative measure.

Hope is Here for Many, but Anxiety Remains

You're not alone if you're feeling uncertain about the future. As the world started to heal from the pandemic, the last restrictions were lifted, and a new post-pandemic world began to evolve, many anticipated an immediate boost in their mental well-being. Yet, a 2022 survey by MIND highlights a shared concern: nearly half of its respondents admitted feeling heightened anxiety about transitions, significant life changes, and upcoming uncertainties. You might resonate with this, especially if you're a young person, as a staggering 91% have expressed facing increased mental challenges since the pandemic's onset. It's okay to feel this way, and understanding these shared experiences can be the first step toward healing and support.

Coronavirus Has Heightened Inequality and Distrust

Before the pandemic, you might have been acutely aware of issues like poverty, mental health challenges, and societal inequalities. Perhaps you even felt their weight in your own life. The pandemic, for many, amplified these disparities, deepening political and social chasms. It's understandable if you found yourself in the midst of heated debates about the reality of COVID-19 or the pros and cons of vaccines. Fueled by deep emotions and concerns, such discussions could easily strain relationships, sometimes pushing loved ones or acquaintances into seemingly opposing camps. It's natural to feel the sadness of those growing distances, especially when they involve close friends, family, or your wider community. Remember, it's a challenging time for all, and every individual's journey and understanding are unique.

"Growing up in a divided family, I gained a unique perspective on the world. One thing that stood out to me was the fraying fabric of the family unit. The lockdown during the pandemic highlighted an unsettling realization for many long-term partners: their lives had become different from what they once knew, and the love they had built together seemed to diminish. It made me question whether these relationships were truly based on genuine love or merely ego-driven. Furthermore, families began

to distance themselves from each other, driven by differing beliefs and fueled by fear. This raises the question of whether the collective consciousness has been further fractured, causing a breakdown in trust and understanding between loved ones. Has the pandemic eroded core values of honor, respect, and integrity?"

Young People Are Finding It Harder to Cope

Research indicates that unhealthy coping mechanisms, such as self-harm or substance abuse, are increasingly prevalent among individuals in the youngest age groups, even more so than adults. It's understandable. With concerns about future careers, education, family, and friends, this age group faces unique challenges. The impact of prolonged isolation and limited social interactions weighs heavily on young people.

"Conversations I've had with many young people reflect the struggles of online learning, the heartache of missing out on milestone celebrations like graduation, and the disheartening loss of enthusiasm for education."

Some have even reconsidered their decision to attend college after all these upheavals. It's deeply distressing, and your feelings are valid if these experiences resonate with you. Remember, you're not alone in this, and together, we can find ways to rebuild that passion for learning and growth. *"Become an entrepreneur and never stop learning."*

People Urgently Need More Support

You deserve more than just basic mental health services. There's still much to be done to ensure that you and others, especially those from racialized and marginalized communities or those facing financial hardships, can access the necessary support to find a wholesome balance in life. Everyone, including you, deserves understanding, compassion, and the resources to thrive.

"Taking responsibility for yourself is the most important step towards healing. Stand up, be heard, and focus!"

RELATABLE STORIES

The profound effects the COVID-19 pandemic has brought to everyone have been extensively discussed. Below are a few real stories that have been documented to offer a glimpse into the world's reality.

- One individual expressed, "I was already in therapy at the start of the pandemic, but I'm going to need a lot more now. The stress, the anxiety, and the isolation—I'm probably at my lowest I've ever been in life right now," (Origanum-majorana, 2022).
- Another shared, "After high school, I was so excited to experience college life, but now I just feel so hopeless. I don't like the quality of knowledge I received from online classes, and I don't even know if all these studies are worth it. I'm not sure if I still have a future or if I can afford what's in the future," (lass_lad, 2022).
- A statement from an expatriate family reads, "Being expats, it was hard for us, not being able to see our family

for two years. We had our second child in 2020, and since then, we can't plan anything! It feels like our lives are at a standstill—we can't move forward," (Anonymous, 2022).

NAVIGATING THE NEW NORMAL: ADAPTING TO CHANGE

From your perspective, there might be doubts about the long-awaited "change" or return to the normalcy everyone yearned for. The world has shifted in unimaginable ways in a short span. It could be important for you to acknowledge that the COVID-19 virus might remain a part of our reality. Research indicates that "COVID-19 is here to stay" and is likely a consistent risk factor among other respiratory viral infections (Emanuel et al., 2022). Yet, it's heartening to see that media attention on the issue has decreased at the time of this writing.

Like others, your desire is for a safe, healthy, and fulfilling life. This current landscape prompts a need for adaptation and resilience. In the following section, let's explore understanding this **"new normal"** and discovering compassionate strategies to navigate these life shifts.

What Does the New Normal Look Like?

As you navigate the new normal, it's evident that each nation and culture has its own unique response to the pandemic's aftermath. You've undoubtedly felt the ripple effects in your daily life, witnessing changes that were once foreign but now routine. Even now, you encounter individuals wearing masks, and at times, some may hesitate to share an elevator with you, still wary of the virus. You might experience this caution on a weekly basis. It's a testament to the deep-seated fears many still harbor. Yet, you respect their defenses with understanding and empathy and adapt with compassion.

Workplace

In this "new normal," you've adapted and reshaped your behaviors, ways of communicating, and how you handle everyday situations with resilience and care. Now, when you feel even the slightest cold or flu symptoms, like a sneeze or fever, you graciously prioritize the well-being of others by staying home until you're back to full health, one thing the pandemic has possibly instilled, self-care. It's a shift from the past when you might have worked through the common cold.

Moreover, there might still be moments when you'll find comfort in using personal protective equipment (PPE) like masks and hand sanitizers, understanding that clean hands do more than just keep you safe; they protect everyone. As you navigate this evolving landscape, remember that these measures, though gradually lessening, are a testament to your commitment to safeguarding yourself and the community around you in these transformative times.

Before the pandemic, the idea of working from home might have felt foreign to you. Perhaps the term "hybrid culture," blending both online and offline work, seemed like a distant concept. Yet, with the pandemic's onset, your professional world underwent a transformation. It's possible you're now among the 71% of employees embracing remote work (Miles, 2022). Maybe you've found solace in the flexibility that hybrid working offers, enabling a more balanced life.

Your employer seems to be recognizing these evolving needs, leaning into flexible schedules that empower you with more autonomy. Now, the global workspace welcomes not only you but people from all walks of life. For those with physical disabilities, the barriers to entry into the workforce might be lowered. If you've been caring for your family at home, this shift might be a beacon, opening avenues for you to contribute while still being present for your loved ones. This evolving work culture, emphasizing inclusivity and diversity, holds promise not just for you but for the world at large, potentially revitalizing the global economy. The beauty of this transformation? You might need a reliable WIFI connection now, and the world becomes your office.

However, let's not forget those impacted differently. The real estate developers, who once thrived on leasing office spaces, are now grappling with a changing landscape. In this new world, while there's much to celebrate, it's essential to approach every change with understanding and empathy.

The New Normal and Mental Health

As you reflect on the aftermath of the pandemic, it's evident that mental health has emerged as a central concern. A survey from the American Psychological Association in 2021 might surprise you: a staggering 84% of psychologists observed a surge in demand for treatments related to anxiety and depressive disorders since the pandemic's onset in 2020. There's also been a marked increase in treatments for conditions like obsessive-compulsive disorders, substance-related disorders, and sleep disturbances. It's a poignant reminder of the profound emotional toll these times have taken.

Recognizing these shifts, it's essential to remember that you're not alone in this journey. If you or your loved ones are grappling with these feelings, it's okay to seek help. The silver lining? The shadows of mental health stigma are fading. There's an ever-growing acceptance and understanding, and now, more than ever, individuals like you are reaching out for support. Whether it's online consultations or other resources, the avenues for help are expanding. Know that it's a sign of strength to seek assistance, and the world is becoming a more understanding place to embrace it. Remember, you are loved, and there's always a helping hand ready to guide you through.

"Don't confine yourself as I once did, yearning for acceptance while grappling with anxiety that only magnified my fears."

CHALLENGES OF ADAPTING TO THE NEW NORMAL AND WHAT TO DO

Navigating changes can be daunting; after all, change is uncomfortable. In facing the new normal, there are countless adjustments you might find yourself grappling with. It's completely natural to feel overwhelmed by such a swift transformation in your day-to-day life. Remember, it's okay to take it one step at a time and seek support when needed. You're not alone on this journey.

So, how exactly can you adapt to this new situation?

Cultivate Critical Thinking Skills

During these trying times, it's essential for you to harness the power of critical thinking. This means cultivating the ability to think clearly, rationally, and objectively, especially when faced with the barrage of information surrounding worldwide changes. Engaging in critical thinking allows you to analyze and evaluate issues before making informed judgments.

Let's explore how you can strengthen this crucial skill:

1. **Analysis:** When you're presented with a flood of new or old pandemic-related information, try breaking it down into simpler parts. This will help you better grasp its essence and significance.
2. **Interpretation:** Aim to truly understand and explain the meaning of data, events, or news about the situation or pandemic.
3. **Evaluation:** Assess the credibility of statements or claims you come across. Are they from reputable sources? Does the evidence support them?
4. **Inference:** From the information at hand, what can you conclude? Ensure your conclusions are grounded in relevant and valid data.

5. **Explanation:** When discussing your views or understanding, strive to articulate your reasoning clearly and concisely.
6. **Self-Regulation:** Take moments to reflect upon your beliefs and understanding about the pandemic. Are there areas where you need to adjust your thinking?
7. **Problem-Solving:** Approach pandemic-related challenges methodically, thinking about potential solutions in a structured way.
8. **Decision Making:** Make choices based on solid reasoning and accurate data, especially when they relate to your health and well-being.

As you nurture your critical thinking mindset, it's compassionate to:

- **Stay Open-minded:** Understand that, especially during such unprecedented times, you might need to change your mind when presented with new evidence or perspectives.
- **Practice Skepticism:** Question ideas and claims. Ensure you have ample evidence before making judgments or decisions.
- **Think for Yourself:** Formulate opinions based on your thorough evaluations, not just what might be trending or popular; that's *the easy way out, yet not always safe.*
- **Recognize Biases:** We all have them. Be aware of your personal biases and try to see beyond them to gain a balanced view. *"Listen to understand, not to respond."*

- **Pursue Truth:** Aim to align your judgments as closely as possible with reality, even if it's sometimes uncomfortable. *"You truly don't understand someone until you've walked in their shoes."*

Critical thinking is more than just a skill; it's a beacon during the fog of uncertainty. By embracing this mindset during any anxious moments, you empower yourself to make informed decisions, foster understanding, and navigate challenges with resilience and clarity. Remember, it's okay to seek help or lean on trusted sources but always do so with an inquisitive and discerning mind.

Create a New Routine

When navigating the world of remote work or adjusting to a home-based role, showing yourself kindness and patience is essential. Crafting a consistent, nurturing routine can be a cornerstone of self-care, helping you bring order to your day. Perhaps setting gentle reminders or alarms could encourage a balanced rhythm. You might choose moments in your day for nourishing meals, focused work, or even brief pockets of relaxation. Remember, you don't need to isolate yourself from your cherished bonds with friends and family. The post-pandemic times might challenge the conventional ways of connection, but they also open doors to creative and meaningful interactions. In this evolving landscape, show yourself the compassion you deserve, knowing you're doing your best.

Focus on Your Motivation

If you find yourself constantly driven by looming deadlines and the anxiety of potential repercussions from unfinished tasks, it might be time to consider a gentler, more compassionate approach to motivation. Instead of being weighed down by stressors, why not highlight the small victories and achievements along the way? Consider crafting a daily to-do list. This simple act can help you remain centered and motivated, allowing you to relish the satisfaction of ticking off completed tasks. Remember, it's not solely about completing the task but recognizing and cherishing each step you take forward. Embracing this method, you'll likely discover that these positive affirmations foster a more nurturing and fulfilling work environment. Every task you complete is a testament to your commitment and efficiency—a small but significant celebration of your journey.

"Create your small victory checklist with one item or ten; when it's completed, check it off, and say, Tada Done!" Celebrate your small accomplishments!

Create a Space for Yourself – Me Time

Have you recognized the importance of self-care for your well-being, especially when striving for productivity or seeking balance in life? Sometimes, you might need that extra moment just for yourself. If you find navigating your emotions or challenges difficult, remember it's okay to seek guidance from a life coach or counselor. Commit to eating on time, ensuring you rest adequately, and prioritizing self-care—an often overlooked step.

Engaging in your favorite hobbies and maintaining a journal to reflect on your emotions can be therapeutic. By embracing these practices, you're setting clear boundaries between work, family, and personal time, showing yourself the compassion you deserve.

At the end of Chapter 8, we've included a daily check-in sheet for you.

THE IMPORTANCE OF MINDSET

Is your glass half-full or half-empty? This age-old question prompts you to reflect on your perspective and how you view the world around you. It highlights that your mindset is indeed a potent instrument. Your mindset, shaped by personal beliefs and perceptions, deeply affects your thoughts, feelings, and actions across various scenarios. How you perceive yourself and the events in your life might be strikingly different from how others see them. Do you see situations as stepping stones or setbacks? *A lot hinges on the faith you place in yourself.*

In this section, you'll explore the significance of mindset. Together, we'll understand how nurturing a resilient mindset can be your guiding light, especially as you adapt to the "new normal" in the wake of the pandemic and other global calamities. Remember, in this journey; every step forward, no matter how small, is progress.

What Is Mindset?

Stanford psychologist Carol Dweck introduced a concept that might deeply resonate with you. According to Dweck, you can possess one of two essential mindsets: fixed or growth. This idea isn't just about whether you see the glass as half-full or half-empty; how you view that glass can reveal a lot about how you interpret your world and experiences.

Developing your mindset helps you make sense of your surroundings and set personal expectations. You might sometimes feel that the new normal is bleak, that the unfolding events are leading to a downward spiral. Such beliefs might make you brace for the worst, diminishing your hope for tomorrow. It's essential to understand that clinging to such a viewpoint can be self-limiting. It might pave the way for feelings of anxiety or sadness, impacting your relationships and overall well-being. Awareness of your mindset is crucial, as it plays a vital role in shaping your mental and emotional health.

"A mindset refers to a set of beliefs and attitudes that shape how an individual perceives and responds to experiences, challenges, and opportunities. It forms the foundation of one's thoughts, behaviors, and overall perspective on life."

So, how do these mindsets differ, and why should you care about their impact on your life?

Fixed Mindset

Those with fixed mindsets often feel that traits, intelligence, or talents are set in stone and unalterable. While there might be a hint of truth in this, it can become harmful if it holds you back from seeking growth and betterment. You might start to believe that success comes only from natural gifts rather than the fruits of persistence and hard work. For instance, you might feel a certain job role is out of reach and decide not to pursue it. By viewing things this way, you might unknowingly cap your potential, preventing the growth you deserve. This can lead to what many call the daunting *"limiting belief."* Remember, everyone has the capacity for growth; it's all about giving yourself a chance to discover it.

Growth Mindset

With a growth mindset, you recognize the boundless potential within yourself. Embracing every new experience and idea, you see challenges not as obstacles but as opportunities for growth. Instead of thinking you're limited by "fixed" abilities, you understand that skills can be nurtured and refined with dedication and heart. When you reflect on your capabilities, you kindly remind yourself, "I may not excel at painting at this moment, but with time and effort, I'll grow and improve." This compassionate and growth-oriented mindset gives you the courage and positivity to face any hurdle, confident in your ever-evolving abilities.

Why Is a Good Mindset Important?

A positive mindset is essential for your growth and ability to face fresh challenges. Understand that no hurdle is too high, and there's always a moment and space for you to evolve. With a robust, hopeful perspective, you can value your progress and stay open to chances that might have otherwise passed you by. Embrace the power of the word "yet" in your daily life. When you face a challenge or a task feels overwhelming, remind yourself that you haven't mastered it "yet." Integrating this simple word into your language can arm you with resilience, ensuring you're always poised to learn and flourish.

Remember, your skills, knowledge, and beliefs aren't set in stone; they can evolve and transform. Take moments to reflect, recognizing your strengths and areas of growth. By understanding yourself more deeply, you empower continuous transformation and betterment.

Embrace the thought: *"Every day, in every way, I'm getting better and better."* Hold that sentiment close to your heart, and **repeat** it **to yourself as you doze off to sleep.**

THE B. B.R.A.V.E. FRAMEWORK

Embracing a positive mindset is vital as you navigate the uncertainties of the post-pandemic world. This book is crafted especially for you, offering a structured approach to help you adopt a growth mindset. By following this path, you can experience the same confidence, peace, and resilience that many others, including the author, have embraced.

Finding optimism requires following these simple steps:

- **B**: Banishing Fear, Worry, and Anxiety with a New Perspective
- **B**: Breaking Negative Thought Patterns
- **R**: Revising Core Beliefs
- **A**: Adopting Mindfulness
- **V**: Vanquishing Procrastination
- **E**: Embracing Sustainable Growth and Thriving

Our discussions on past pandemics might have stirred feelings of anxiety or discomfort, but it's essential to recognize that by addressing these topics, we pave the way for understanding and adjusting to our current reality. Embracing and adapting to the new normal is a testament to our resilience and progress.

The importance of mental well-being in maintaining a healthy and fulfilling life has been emphasized, and the urgent need for support in the post-pandemic era is clear. It becomes essential to adopt a new lifestyle promoting self-growth.

The next step involves **banishing fear, worry, and anxiety, replacing them with a new perspective.**

"Always place your becoming above your current being."

— DR. JORDAN B. PETERSON

2

BANISHING FEAR, WORRY, AND ANXIETY WITH A NEW PERSPECTIVE

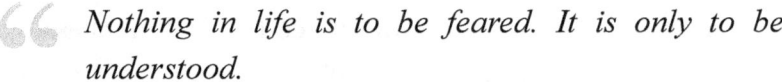 *Nothing in life is to be feared. It is only to be understood.*

Life moves forward, and you persevere, drawing from an intrinsic capability to face fears head-on. Consider for a moment your experiences, like soaring in an airplane high above the earth. Just a few centuries back, wouldn't such an act have seemed unearthly, perhaps even magical to you? Yet, because of the audacity and courage of people in the past, you've seen advancements like air travel become a reality. Just as humanity pushes boundaries by tackling its collective fears, you can grow immensely by addressing your personal anxieties.

Fears, uncertainties, and worries are integral to your journey. They emerge when you're poised at the brink of challenges or novel situations. These emotions are deep-rooted, coursing through both your conscious and subconscious mind. They play a pivotal role in shaping your self-awareness and carving out your unique identity. Your emotions emphasize the richness and singularity of your life's tapestry.

Perhaps, like many, you've found yourself sidestepping distressing situations that rouse unease or trigger that intrinsic fight, flight or freeze response in you. While such moments can be jarring, they also serve as stark reminders of your human vulnerability and, at the same time, your remarkable resilience. Recognize that your growth emerges from acknowledging and embracing these uneasy moments. It's in these spaces of discomfort that you genuinely evolve.

When you view your emotions with a heart full of compassion, they take on a pivotal role in your life's journey. They inspire, shape, and deepen your empathy. Choosing to approach these feelings with kindness and understanding unlocks a world of growth. Without confronting these challenges head-on, there's a possibility that the vast landscapes of personal growth remain uncharted.

For the sake of mental well-being, it's crucial for you to acknowledge, allow and confront any negative emotions. To sidestep them is to bypass invaluable opportunities for self-improvement. Imagine letting a lingering fear of flying tether you from your dream of piloting an aircraft. To transcend this obstacle, start by recognizing your fear and working diligently to overcome it. In the coming sections, I'll guide you in forging strategies to navigate through your fears, worries, and anxieties.

The objective isn't to shove these fears into the shadows but to embrace them as facets of your being. This acceptance cultivates resilience and self-assurance, empowering you to adapt to life's ever-shifting sands. Together, we'll discover coping techniques that help reframe these challenges, viewing them not as hindrances but as stepping stones to personal growth. Let's remember: your anxieties are natural, and through tools like mindfulness, they can be channeled into pathways of enlightenment and self-understanding.

You can face challenges with a renewed mindset by recognizing your negative emotions and seeing them as opportunities for personal growth. This approach enables you to nurture empathy and compassion within yourself.

This is my application of the first **'B' in the B-BRAVE framework**.

Developing Coping Strategies for Fear, Worry, and Codependency

To confront your fears, concerns, and anxieties, you first need to understand how they form in your consciousness—how they mold your thoughts, sway your actions, and how they manifest psychologically. It's crucial for you to discern patterns in your thinking, especially those emotional triggers. For example, when a certain word or phrase makes you suddenly uneasy, those are the telltale signs you should be attuned to. Acknowledging these cues is essential in identifying the sources of your anxieties and fears, laying the groundwork to face them head-on.

Imagine attending a workshop on **Codependency**, and during a session, a counselor remarks on something as trivial as you not wearing a name tag. Such a seemingly inconsequential comment from someone in a position of authority can stir up feelings of anxiety and unease. But what if, at that moment, you were fully present, able to swiftly recognize this emotional surge and trace it back to an event from your past? That kind of mindfulness and acute awareness can be a beacon for healing.

In previous instances, similar situations might have engulfed you. You could have felt trapped in a fog of apprehension, there in body but distant in spirit, burdened by the overwhelming nature of those emotions.

As you continue on this journey, it's pivotal to understand and address aspects like codependency. Workshops and counseling sessions can indeed shed light on your "inner child." This term pertains to your younger self, particularly during the ages of 0 to 8. As noted by organizations like the Centers for Disease Control and Prevention, events during these foundational years, be they joyous or traumatic, play a significant role in shaping one's development, casting long shadows into adulthood.

Let's together embark on a journey toward inner peace, personal empowerment, and a rejuvenated sense of liberation.

"It was my name tag that was missing."

WHAT IS CODEPENDENCY?

Codependency is a multifaceted emotional and behavioral state that can influence your ability to cultivate balanced, reciprocal relationships. It often manifests as a profound reliance on others for validation and a sense of personal identity. Such feelings can trace back to early years when you might have adjusted or modified your behavior to maneuver through a difficult or unpredictable environment, perhaps due to an unstable family setting.

When you're in a relationship influenced by codependency, you might consistently place another's needs above your own, sometimes neglecting your own emotional health and well-being. This can even result in unintentionally encouraging the other person's detrimental habits, fitting the mold of an ever-accommodating people pleaser.

It's not rare for those grappling with codependency to wrestle with sensations of guilt, feelings of diminished self-worth, and challenges in nurturing self-love. This can stem from seeking an identity in others rather than fostering a confident and loving relationship with oneself.

Reflecting on your personal experiences, you might identify that feelings of abandonment in your formative years influenced your deep-seated desire to maintain equilibrium, often suppressing your own emotions to ensure peace within the family dynamic.

Considering challenges like your father's absence and the trials faced by a single mother raising three sons, it's understandable if you adopted a pattern of prioritizing others' well-being over your own.

It's paramount to recognize that conditions like codependency aren't indictments of personal failures but are responses to complex circumstances. With heightened self-awareness, compassion, and expert advice, these challenges can be acknowledged and addressed, leading to a path of healing and growth.

Here is a brief outline of topics covered in a codependency workshop:

- Am I codependent?
- Symptoms of codependency
- Creating a bond of trust – Trust & Self Disclosure
- Understanding Feelings, *not how are you,* but how you are feeling
- JOHARI – Window of Self
- Understanding Self Esteem
- Rational Self Counseling – Rational vs Irrational Thinking
- AL-ANONS 12 Steps
- Defense Mechanisms
- Progression and Recovery
- Family Communication
- Detach from Damaging Relationships
- Assertive Formula
- Every Person's Bill of Rights – Referenced below
- Anger Management Awareness
- Kissing Guilt and Shame Goodbye

- Daily Morning Check-ins cover how you feel physically, mentally, emotionally, and spiritually; meditation is a great exercise at the back of the book.

Next, you'll discover techniques to counteract these challenging emotions. Beyond embracing mindfulness and self-compassion, consider surrounding yourself with a strong support network or even seeking professional guidance. This will bolster your courage and resilience. The path ahead is for you to cultivate a life filled with inner joy, profound strength, and a renewed sense of freedom. Remember, taking these steps in this journey showcases immense bravery and self-care.

JOHARI – Window of Self

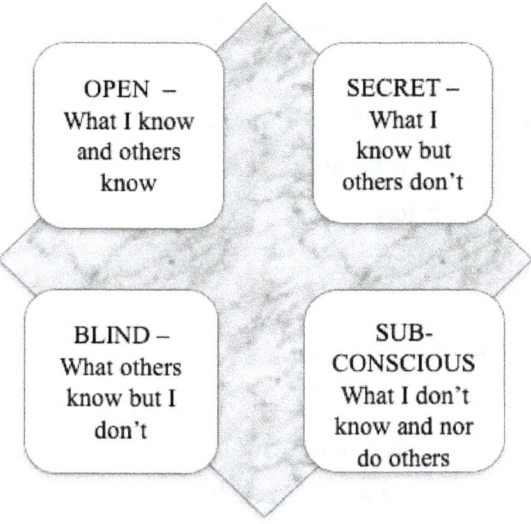

EVERY PERSON'S BILL OF RIGHTS

- The right to be treated with respect.
- The right to have and express your own feelings and opinions.
- The right to be listened to and taken seriously.
- The right to set your own priorities.
- The right to say no without feeling guilty.
- The right to ask for what you want.
- The right to ask for information from professionals.
- The right to make mistakes.
- The right to get what you pay for.
- The right to choose not to assert yourself.
- The right to change your mind.
- The right to say: "I don't know the answer."
- The right to say: "I need some time to think that over."
- The right to add to your bill of rights.
- I have the right to expect honesty from others.
- I have the right to be angry at someone I love.
- I have the right to be uniquely myself.
- How to be assertive in specific situations.

The Nature of Codependency

You may often feel caught in a loop, consistently prioritizing the needs of others over your own. Always striving to make those around you happy, you might inadvertently put your own needs on the back burner. Do you sometimes feel like you're carrying the weight of others' emotions? Does setting personal boundaries seem almost impossible? This could be a sign of codependency, a situation where the line between your needs and those of others becomes blurred. While it's commendable to be compassionate and selfless, there's a fine line between genuinely helping others and neglecting oneself.

You might see these tendencies as just being kind-hearted, and it's beautiful to have such a giving nature. However, it's essential to remember that your well-being is equally important. Ensuring you have healthy boundaries is a crucial step towards experiencing a fulfilling life where you're not constantly burdened by the weight of everyone else's emotions and actions.

If any of this sounds familiar, you might want to delve deeper into understanding the origins of codependency and discover ways to navigate and heal. Remember, it's not just about caring for others; it's about caring for yourself too.

"In my workshop, I had an enlightening moment where I recognized numerous patterns I had developed over time as defense mechanisms. For instance, whenever I conceived a promising business idea, I would eagerly share it with a friend. But upon reflection, I wasn't necessarily looking to pursue the idea; rather, I was seeking external validation. This thrill of having someone else appreciate my concept was actually a way to soothe the deep-seated feelings of abandonment from my childhood, stemming from issues with my parent's divorce.

"As a recovering codependent, I now jot down these ideas. I reflect on them to determine whether I can capitalize on them or

set them aside, as they might not address a genuine need for the consumer."

How Anxiety Fuels Codependency

Anxiety can sometimes feel like a heavy burden on your shoulders, affecting not only your actions but also your relationships with those close to you. It's completely natural for you to want to retreat and find comfort in solitude, especially during moments when anxiety feels all-consuming. There might be times when you crave consistency and understanding from those you love, getting so wrapped up in your emotions that you might momentarily forget the mutual exchange that sustains strong bonds.

On the other hand, perhaps your anxiety stems from a profound sense of care for those around you. Such intense feelings can occasionally lead you to be overly protective or doubtful, unintentionally casting a shadow of uncertainty or hyper-awareness over your interactions.

It's important to know that reaching out for support is a sign of strength, not weakness. Yet, it's equally vital to ensure that your relationships maintain a sense of balance. Anxiety has a way of making one lean heavily on others through a need for another's validation or assurance. But trust in your inner resilience to confront and manage these anxious waves. And remember, true connections are always rooted in mutual respect, understanding, and growth.

"Experiencing anxiety has been a significant challenge for me. I recall the intensity of my first major anxiety attack and how

debilitating it felt. The overwhelming sensations clouded my mind, impacting my relationships significantly. If I wasn't careful, or if I wasn't in the moment and self-aware, I would unknowingly sabotage my connections. I took my mother's advice to heart at an early age: you show more contempt by saying nothing. Therefore, I often kept silent when someone said something hurtful. I internalized that pain, allowing it to fester into resentment. Before I knew it, my instinct to distance myself or cut ties with those individuals took over. It was my way of seeking refuge; it was flight mode."

Ways to Overcome Codependency

Firstly, it's important to recognize the truth within yourself. Like many, you might be unaware of your codependent tendencies. Leaving the comfort of familiar relationships, even if dysfunctional, can feel overwhelming. Yet, recognizing and naming these feelings is the very beginning of your path to healing. Allow yourself to sit with these emotions; they hold the potential to guide you toward more wholesome relationships with others, especially yourself.

Taking a step further, consider reflecting on relationships from your past and present. Identifying any past events or experiences that contribute to your codependency can be illuminating. Remember, it's completely okay if this introspection brings up difficult feelings. You don't have to walk this path alone; consider seeking the guidance of a trusted therapist or a supportive group who can truly understand and empathize with your journey.

As you move forward, think about which relationships truly uplift you and which might be hindering your growth. Your well-being should be a priority, and this means centering yourself and your needs. It's a gentle reminder that you aren't solely responsible for someone else's happiness. Sometimes, letting go of the urge to control every situation and understanding where your limits lie can bring immense peace.

Additionally, consider the power of saying "no." It might feel challenging initially, especially if you're accustomed to placing others' needs above yours. Let's say you've had a long week and are looking forward to some quiet time, but then a friend asks for your help. It's entirely okay to prioritize your rest. Some might be taken aback by this newfound assertion, but genuine friendships will always respect your boundaries. If these steps feel daunting, please remember you're not alone. Professional guidance or support groups dedicated to codependency can offer invaluable insights and support.

"The start of my initial dysfunctional relationship coincided with the onset of COVID. I found myself strongly leaning into my codependent tendencies, desperately trying to mend things, holding onto the belief that "we can work through this." Yet, my partner was steadily drifting away, leaving me fearing yet another loss. I proposed counseling as a solution, but she declined, suggesting I'd only blame her throughout the process. It was then that I realized she had been manipulating and gaslighting me throughout our relationship. As someone constantly fearful of losing love and connection, I overlooked the most crucial person in my life: myself. At that moment, I wasn't

familiar with the term "narcissist," but I was living that reality. Nonetheless, I'm thankful for the experience. It taught me about boundaries, the true essence of love, and, most importantly, how to love myself. Even though growth often emerges from profound pain, when engulfed in confusion, I've learned to take a step back, breathe, meditate, focus, and prioritize self-love."

HOW TO OVERCOME FEAR AND ANXIETY

At times, you might find yourself wrestling with fear and anxiety. It's completely natural, and everyone feels this way occasionally. However, sometimes these emotions can become overwhelming, making it hard for you to sort through your thoughts. As you may recall, many people instinctively react with a flight, fight, or freeze response, trying to distance themselves from whatever is causing distress. Some individuals face heightened levels of fear due to conditions like anxiety disorder, panic disorder, or specific phobias, which can profoundly impact one's well-being.

While it's common to feel fear and anxiety simultaneously, understanding their subtle differences can offer clarity about your emotional state. Equipped with this knowledge and certain coping strategies, you'll be better positioned to navigate these feelings with compassion and understanding for yourself.

Understanding the Difference Between Fear and Anxiety

To understand the difference:

Anxiety is the anticipation of a future threat, often manifesting in prolonged worry, tension, and nervousness about what might happen. It is less tied to a specific, immediate threat and more about future uncertainties.

Common symptoms of anxiety include:

- overthinking
- restlessness
- sleeping problems (either excessively sleeping or sleep-deprived)
- physical and/or emotional fatigue
- difficulty concentrating
- irritability or anger issues
- tense muscles
- digestive issues, usually stemming from poor diet

Fear is an emotional response to an immediate, known, or perceived threat. It is a survival mechanism that triggers the body's "fight, flight-or-freeze" response.

Common signs of fear include:

- increased heart rate
- cold sweat
- shortness of breath
- trembling
- dry mouth
- nausea

You might notice that fear and anxiety often walk hand in hand. For example, living in an area where you don't feel completely safe might bring about a lingering fear, causing you to constantly worry about the possibility of break-ins. These uneasy thoughts can come up again and again, amplifying your anxiety. When you dive deep into understanding them, the distinction between fear and anxiety is mainly about context. Fear springs from a clear and present danger, setting off that immediate fight or flight reaction within you. On the other hand, anxiety might creep up even when there's no direct threat, yet it stirs a similar emotional response. Remember, it's completely natural to feel this way, and understanding these emotions can be the first step towards addressing them with compassion and care.

TECHNIQUES TO TREAT ANXIETY

Under various situations, you might find it beneficial to seek the guidance of a professional therapist or a support group. Many find connecting with others who understand their struggles incredibly relieving, almost like finding a second family.

Engaging with a counselor can offer you invaluable insights into your mental well-being and introduce you to therapeutic methods tailored to your needs. Some therapists, depending on their specialization, might be able to provide a medical diagnosis for any concerns you have. And if they're not the right fit, they're usually well-connected to guide you toward further specialized diagnostic or medical assistance.

For those feeling the weight of anxiety, therapies like cognitive behavioral therapy (CBT), acceptance and commitment therapy (ACT), emotional freedom techniques, and emotion-focused therapy are often explored. Remember, there's a world of support out there, waiting to help you navigate your feelings with care and understanding.

Cognitive Behavioral Therapy

CBT invites you, through the embrace of mindfulness, to reshape or reframe any distorted thoughts that may be holding you back. Your therapist aims to help you identify thought patterns that may be causing you distress. It's common with anxiety to sometimes slip into unhelpful ways of thinking, like assuming the worst or focusing excessively on negative outcomes. In therapy, you'll be gently encouraged to observe and reflect on these thoughts, confront situations that might heighten your anxiety, and work collaboratively on problem-solving. Through this, you'll cultivate a deeper understanding of your anxiety, enhance your ability to assess situations, and grow more confident in navigating life's complexities. Remember, this journey is about understanding yourself better and empowering you to live a life with greater ease and understanding.

Acceptance and Commitment Therapy

ACT is a form of mindfulness therapy that can help you foster psychological flexibility and mental resilience. This compassionate approach recognizes the struggles you've faced and invites you to confront challenges and fully feel your emotions, even when they're painful. You're then guided to adopt proactive strategies, focusing on a hopeful future instead of getting trapped in past regrets. By consistently moving forward with resilience, despite life's hurdles, you have the potential to break free from long-standing negative thought cycles, paving the way for more positive mental well-being.

Emotional Freedom Techniques

In Chinese medicine, there's a gentle technique often called "tapping" or "psychological acupressure" that you might find comforting. Imagine a self-soothing method where you gently tap specific acupressure points with your fingers, all while focusing on a particular concern or emotion. It's reminiscent of acupuncture, but the touch of your own fingertips replaces needles. By engaging these meridian points, you have the potential to alleviate stress and find emotional balance. When you're navigating those moments of overwhelm, consider embracing this method as a way to show yourself some kindness and care.

Emotion-Focused Therapy

This approach understands that your emotions deeply influence your identity. It encourages you to honor and trust your emotions, letting them steer you toward meaningful and intentional choices in life—listening to that inner voice or gut feeling. A compassionate therapist can guide you to connect more profoundly with your feelings, show you how to navigate them and assist you in expressing them authentically. Through this method, you're empowered to reshape your negative emotions, create nurturing coping strategies, and develop personal habits to address and rise above counterproductive thoughts. It's all about discerning rational from irrational thinking.

TIPS TO OVERCOME FEAR AND ANXIETY

You're not alone in facing anxiety, and it's commendable that you're seeking ways to navigate it. Beyond professional therapy, which is a valuable resource, there are various methods you might find comforting. Let's explore some activities and practices together, gently guiding you toward a space of ease and clarity. Remember, it's about finding what resonates with you and taking one step at a time.

Consider Yoga

Yoga presents a unique opportunity for you. By synchronizing your breath with the gentle rhythms of your body, you can achieve a harmonious balance between mind and movement. When you immerse yourself in yoga, you're not just engaging in physical exercise but also embracing spiritual and mental disciplines. This holistic practice can be a soothing balm for your soul, ushering in peace and inner calm. Moreover, intertwining yoga with psychotherapy can be a transformative experience for you. Research suggests that when you incorporate yoga into your routine, it can help alleviate anxiety and depression symptoms, offering a supportive hand in managing panic disorders (Saeed et al., 2019). Remember, this journey is yours, and yoga can be a compassionate companion along the way.

Soma Breathwork

You might have heard of Niraj Naik, often referred to as The Renegade Pharmacist. He developed Soma breathwork, a special breathing and meditation technique tailored just for individuals like you. By combining rhythmic breathing patterns with visualization and unique breath retention methods, this approach is designed with care to guide you toward relaxation, balance, and personal evolution. Embrace it, and let it be a compassionate tool to aid your journey toward well-being.

"From my journey, I've found solace and healing in yoga and breathwork. These practices have been my refuge, guiding me through anxiety and leading me toward a profound inner peace.

With each pose and every mindful breath, I've embraced a more profound sense of grace and honor."

Limit or Avoid Caffeine Intake

As you take a moment to consider your well-being, it's worth noting the effects of caffeine, commonly found in chocolate, coffee, and tea. Remember, while many enjoy their daily caffeine fix without issue, it might not be the best for everyone. Overconsumption can exacerbate anxiety and disrupt restful sleep, as pointed out by a study by Temple et al. (2017). If you've been feeling anxious, perhaps consider reducing your intake, maybe to just a single morning cup or even taking a break from it altogether. Always prioritize what feels right for your body and mind.

"The first time I experienced an anxiety attack, I ended up in the hospital, genuinely believing I was suffering from a heart attack. The doctor who saw me explained the primary triggers for anxiety, highlighting caffeine as a top culprit."

Practice Mindfulness Meditation

Just as yoga offers you solace and strength, meditation might bring a profound sense of healing to your soul. When you center your attention on each breath, every fleeting emotion, and the subtle sensations of the present moment through mindfulness meditation, you're truly connecting with your inner self. This practice invites you to embrace the present, nurturing a deeper understanding and compassion for yourself.

"When I began meditating, I initially believed it wouldn't benefit me, a testament to my then-fixed mindset. To counteract this, I embraced a growth mindset to transcend that restrictive belief. Whenever distractions arose, be it a passing car or fleeting thoughts, I homed in on the sound of my breathing to anchor me back to tranquility."

Keep a Journal or Diary

When you find yourself swamped with intense emotions, consider pouring those feelings onto the pages of a notebook or daily diary. Often, the act of writing can help bring clarity to the storm of thoughts swirling within. Should anxiety or fear weigh heavy on your heart, pause for a moment. Write down what you feel and try to understand where it's coming from. This simple act can be a gentle embrace of your emotions, offering a moment of understanding and self-compassion. After writing, read your words aloud. Hear them, feel them. And then, if it feels right, consider erasing them or tearing that page. This symbolic gesture can remind you of your strength and resilience, reassuring you that you've faced your emotions and are prepared to step forward with renewed hope and confidence. This tender approach might be the soothing balm you need, a heartfelt strategy to better connect with and understand your own heart's whisperings.

"Whenever I experience anger or disappointment, I have a ritual that I've always followed. And no, it doesn't involve any voodoo dolls with pins and needles! What I do is grab a pen and paper, and I pour out my emotions. Sometimes I write a letter, and other

times I just jot down my feelings in point form. Once I've transferred all those emotions onto the paper, I burn it. As the flames consume the paper, I tell myself that I'm letting go of these feelings. It's an incredibly freeing experience."*

EMBRACING AND HARNESSING ANXIETY FOR GROWTH AND RESILIENCE

Imagine your anxiety as a fire alarm. It's there for a reason, alerting you to potential concerns—much like an alarm signals a fire. When you acknowledge and address the root cause, the overwhelming feelings can subside, maybe even disappear. But if ignored, it can escalate and become unmanageable.

As a naturally intuitive being, it's vital for you to understand which signals to heed and which to reassess. Armed with the right tools and knowledge, you're more than capable of navigating these feelings. By doing so, you're not only ensuring your well-being but also enriching your life's journey. It's essential to listen, truly listen, to what your inner self is communicating.

In the pages ahead, you'll uncover compassionate ways to understand and guide your anxiety, transforming it from a potential obstacle into a powerful ally.

"I've come to embrace these emotions, seeing them as signals or messages for personal growth and evolution."

Anxiety as the Path to Freedom

When you think about freedom, anxiety might not be the first thing that comes to your mind. It's easy to see anxiety as a foe, something to avoid, especially given the hushed conversations that might occur behind closed doors about someone's mental well-being. But real freedom isn't about living without anxiety or escaping from difficult emotions; it's about your ability to acknowledge, face, and understand them. These emotions are here to help you come to terms with reality. Your vulnerability is like a gentle nudge urging you to look inside and find your truths.

Feeling anxious doesn't make you weak; in fact, it highlights your humanity. It's a testament to your resilience and deep awareness, both crucial to our shared human journey.

You hold within you the strength to turn your anxiety into a path to freedom. By connecting with yourself, you can discern the subtle signs your body is showing you, whether it's a momentary cloudiness in your thoughts or the physical unease you might feel in your tense shoulders or fidgety fingers. Welcome these challenging moments, approach them with an open heart, and bravely step into the unknown. This is your path to emotional growth.

True liberation comes from accepting every part of yourself: your flaws, vulnerabilities, and all the emotions that stir within you. Instead of pushing them away, or trying to silence them, let these feelings move through you. When you truly listen to them, both your mind and body will sense the safe space you've created. Remember, you're deserving of compassion and understanding, always.

"When I feel anxious, I often put my mask on and continue with my tasks. I wonder, am I showing my authentic self, or am I projecting an image I believe society expects of me? Do I become the role, like so many who immerse themselves in their work persona and bring that persona home? Instead of revealing genuine emotions, I sometimes show only the ego-driven version of myself, all for acceptance or inclusion."

"My twenty-first birthday was an emotional time for me. I remember questioning my identity and purpose seeking guidance from my mother, who advised me based on her own level of understanding. She emphasized the importance of being a good provider and finding a reliable job. While I listened to her mentorship, I realized that finding answers to my questions required me to look within myself, which I did briefly then. Despite the challenge of being a male during the Industrial Revolution and the cultural norm of suppressing emotions, I persisted and became stronger in my journey of self-discovery."

WAYS TO USE ANXIETY AS A SOURCE FOR GROWTH

Label It

Throughout your life, you've often felt the push and pull of viewing things in absolutes, as black or white. When negative emotions arise, they've often been signals for you, inviting introspection and understanding. On the other hand, positive emotions have felt like beacons, illuminating your growth and inviting you to embrace and celebrate them. Yet, with time and reflection, you've come to see that emotions don't always fit within these clear-cut boundaries. Feelings like fear, anxiety, and worry are a part of the complex tapestry of your being. They are a gentle reminder that embracing uncertainty and acceptance isn't a new journey but a path you've always been on, one step at a time.

"When a negative thought or belief crosses my mind, I jot it down to tackle it later, depending on my setting—be it at work, a social event, or any other situation. If the moment feels right, I immediately question whether it aligns with my greater purpose."

Address It

When anxiety surfaces within you, it's compassionate to pause and deeply examine the thoughts, sensations, and emotions that accompany it. Ask yourself, "How do you truly experience this?" and "Where in your body do you feel it?" Posing these questions gently invites you to attune and observe. You might notice your thoughts racing or repeating, fostering a sense of restlessness. Physically, there could be a tightening in your chest, a quickened heartbeat, or tension in your muscles. On the emotional front, feelings of apprehension, unease, or general discomfort may arise. Acknowledging and identifying these facets gives you insight into the form anxiety takes within you, empowering you to face it with compassion and implement effective strategies to ease its impact.

"When my body and mind align under the weight of anxiety, I experience a tightness in my chest and a haze over my thoughts, often referred to as brain fog. If I'm mindful and present, this feeling may only last for a brief moment; however, if left unchecked, it can persist for days or even weeks."

Stop Resisting and Embrace Anxiety

Navigating the landscape of your emotions can feel daunting, but there's strength in approaching your anxiety with a sense of curiosity and nurturing self-compassion. Consider reframing how you view emotions, moving away from the rigid dichotomy of "good" versus "bad." Start by acknowledging all feelings, both those that uplift and those that weigh you down. Perhaps on one side of the page, you list feelings of joy, contentment, and fulfillment; on the other, emotions like sorrow, doubt, and fear. It's crucial to allow yourself the space to feel each emotion fully. Engage in a gentle practice of drawing in positive emotions with each breath and releasing the challenging ones as you exhale. This gentle approach encourages acceptance and offers a compassionate way to navigate through the intricacies of your feelings.

"I concealed it when I first discovered that I was grappling with anxiety. I feared judgment; perhaps some might have discerned my struggle and either exploited it or were pushed away by it. This was the irrational part of my mind playing its self-sabotaging tricks. However, by acknowledging these emotions and recognizing their origins, I've gained a sense of liberation that's challenging to articulate—a genuine sense of happiness!"

Break Down Intrusive Thoughts

When you let anxiety linger, it can manifest as intrusive thoughts. These unwelcome musings can distract you from the present, overshadowing the joys of your day. Sometimes, they might even make you believe that your deepest fears are absolute truths. They subtly plant seeds of doubt, preventing you from connecting with your true emotions. Simply trying to ignore or avoid these thoughts isn't the solution; it often gives them even more power. However, there's a gentle way to find some relief. Consider keeping a journal dedicated to these challenging thoughts. Write them down, observe how you feel, and gently remind yourself that they're just distorted reflections of your anxiety. This compassionate approach allows you to understand and navigate these emotions more clearly and kindly.

"One method I have used over the years is practicing **Ho'Oponopono***".*

*"****Ho'oponopono*** *is an ancient Hawaiian practice of reconciliation and forgiveness. The term "Ho'Oponopono" can be translated as "to make right" or "to correct an error." It's a method to restore balance in relationships and within oneself.*

The Ho'oponopono prayer is often summarized by its four simple phrases:

1. *I'm sorry.*
2. *Please forgive me.*
3. *Thank you.*
4. *I love you.*

These phrases are used as a form of mental and spiritual cleansing to rectify any past wrongs or burdens. By reciting them, one acknowledges mistakes, asks for forgiveness, expresses gratitude, and affirms love, seeking to cleanse the heart and mind of negative thoughts or memories. The idea behind the prayer is that taking responsibility for one's actions, thoughts, and feelings can heal and transform negative energies into positive ones."

Learn to Interpret Intrusive Thoughts as Symbols

Once you learn to create a gentle space between yourself and your intrusive thoughts, you can compassionately acknowledge the pain they might bring. Remember, pain is a shared human experience, and it's a part of our journey. Kindly encourage yourself to write down these thoughts, viewing them not as intruders but as messengers pointing to deeper feelings. For instance, if thoughts about your physical appearance emerge, or if envy creeps in when you see others being admired, pause and send love to those emotions. Ask yourself: Are underlying feelings of discontent or unhappiness surfacing? Hold those emotions with care, allow yourself to genuinely experience them, and then gently let them drift away. This gentle approach often leads to more profound insights and healing than continually striving for external validation.

Each time an intrusive or negative thought enters my mind, I recite the Ho'Oponopono Prayer to myself: "I love myself, I apologize, I ask for my own forgiveness, and I express gratitude with thank you."

Check in With Yourself Regularly

Checking in with yourself can be challenging, especially when life gets busy. Amidst the hustle of attending to family needs or meeting work deadlines, it's easy to lose touch with your inner world. Remember, it's crucial to stay connected with your thoughts and feelings, and yes, it requires practice. **Trust me; you're not alone.** I've been their countless times *on* this journey. To help you navigate, consider embracing practices that have benefited many. Set aside moments for self-reflection, maintain a journal, explore mindfulness or meditation, or simply find quiet moments to reconnect with your core. By taking these mindful steps, you'll not only nurture your well-being but also foster a deeper self-awareness, even amidst life's chaos.

"Amidst the overwhelming news and clamor of the pandemic and unfolding events, I felt adrift in numerous aspects of my life, which prompted a stronger resolve to prioritize self-care. Now, I devote an hour every morning to personal growth and self-reflection."

DEVELOP OPTIMISM AND MENTAL RESILIENCE TO CONQUER ANXIETY

Optimism is your guiding light and your protective barrier against unforeseen challenges. It encourages you to find hidden blessings, strengthen your mental fortitude, and approach life's obstacles with an open heart and mind. It's more than just a mindset; optimism becomes your perspective, shaping how you interact with the world. By adopting this hopeful outlook, you foster self-belief, transforming into someone who remains steadfast, even when faced with life's unexpected twists. Remember, everyone faces their share of challenges. With optimism, you'll zero in on the potential for positive outcomes rather than getting lost in a maze of negativity.

During the rise of the COVID-19 pandemic, I felt overwhelmed by the flood of information from the mainstream media and health officials. They talked about new ways of living, the importance of social distancing, and the promise of vaccine safety. My anxiety surged as I tried to navigate these waves of information, which sometimes felt conflicting. As an essential worker, adjusting to the new PPE guidelines drastically altered how I performed my duties. I constantly questioned myself: Was I overreacting? Were the updates indeed for my benefit or causing more harm? Was this heightened anxiety a curse or, in some twisted way, a blessing in disguise?

In this section, I'll share some tips to guide you in cultivating an optimistic mindset, helping you navigate life's roller-coaster with added resilience.

USE THESE TIPS TO INCREASE YOUR MENTAL RESILIENCE

Change Your Narrative

When you encounter obstacles, it's natural to sometimes fixate on the negatives. It can lead you down a path of self-doubt and envision the bleakest scenarios. Remember, you have the power within you to shift this narrative. By embracing positive affirmations, you can nurture optimism and provide yourself with the gentle care and understanding you deserve.

"During the pandemic, I felt like I was constantly on a hamster wheel, trying to figure out the best way to protect myself. It was a natural defense mechanism. I wondered if the government was genuinely trying to help or using the virus to exert control. I questioned whether society had ever taken such measures to prevent the spread of disease before. I'm unsure if these thoughts are pessimistic or optimistic, but I believe we can all shift our perspective and change our narrative."

Learn to Be Grateful

Finding gratitude doesn't always come from grand achievements. You might discover it in the subtle, everyday moments. Think about the quiet yet profound truths: you opened your eyes to a new day and navigated through a global pandemic. You're still standing, ready to treasure times with your loved ones. Hold onto this heartwarming lens of gratitude.

"As I reflected on the best path for me during the pandemic, I recognized my growing gratitude for the clarity of my thoughts and the choices available to me through the rights I hold as a citizen of my country. It is something I must advocate for, not just for my sake but also for my children and grandchildren."

Focus on Things You Can Control

You may often find yourself burdened by the weight of global challenges like the pandemic or the threats of war, climate change, racism, and inequality. It's wholly understandable to seek knowledge and understanding about these issues, but remember, focusing solely on immediate, monumental changes can be draining. Just as the pandemic wasn't resolved in a day, neither will these complex problems. When everyone's energy is absorbed by these vast concerns, it can impact both our collective spirit and our personal well-being. It's crucial for your peace of mind to focus on the aspects you can influence and the steps you can take today. For example, in your journey to support the environment, consider embracing reusable products to minimize waste. Remember, each small step you take is a ripple, and together, these ripples can create waves of lasting change.

"I felt overwhelmed by my downward spiraling anxiety, especially when it came to the health of those around me and the decisions made by elected officials that seemed to infringe on our rights in what's supposed to be a democratic society. My overall well-being was deteriorating, with my usual positive energy and happiness waning, making me feel like a rudderless boat adrift at sea. Eventually, I recognized the toll these uncontrollable

external factors were taking on my mental state. I have always been an optimistic and hardworking individual, facing challenges head-on. Recognizing this, I made a conscious decision to focus on what was within my control and committed to improving my own well-being and raising my vibration to new levels."

Surround Yourself with Optimists

Just like laughter, optimism can resonate deeply within you. It's truly nurturing for you to be in the company of those who align with your dreams, echo your positive outlook, and offer a comforting beam of hope when your spirits need a gentle lift.

"I recently experienced being optimistic again during the codependency workshop I attended. These individuals have become my beacon of optimism, just like many others in my life. It's essential to find your tribe."

Establish Supportive and Positive Relationships

You deserve to surround yourself with individuals or groups who uplift and nurture you. Finding those who radiate positivity and offer genuine encouragement can be a source of solace and strength. It's so important to create and cherish these meaningful connections, allowing you to be your authentic self and drawing comfort from the bonds you share. Remember, nurturing these relationships can be a balm for the soul, especially in challenging times.

"I've been to several support groups to help me navigate my personal challenges. I've personally attended AL-ANON and CODA sessions, and it's been incredibly uplifting to connect with others who understand and share similar life struggles. There's no judgment there, just genuine people sharing their stories, giving me a chance to listen, relate, and learn."

Wake up With a Positive Thought

You start your day with a thought that rejuvenates and drives you. Instead of lamenting the upcoming traffic, you gently remind yourself how fortunate you are to have the health and ability to drive. And even on those rainy mornings, you comfort yourself with the knowledge that the sun is shining brightly somewhere. Such reflections encourage you to appreciate and treasure the present moment, showing kindness to yourself along the way.

"I have adorned my walls with inspirational pictures and quotes."

Engage in Leisure Activities

Your life isn't solely defined by the work you do, and that's true for everyone. It's perfectly okay to embrace activities that nurture your well-being. How about exploring a new hobby or indulging in calming pursuits? Perhaps a peaceful walk in the park, getting lost in your favorite song, or diving deep into a riveting book? All these moments can be gentle ways to ease stress and lift your spirits. Remember, it's not only about doing but also about being and feeling; you deserve every moment of joy and relaxation.

"Leisure activities have always been a challenge for me. As I've shared, my parents divorced, and I took on responsibilities from a young age. As a result, I naturally gravitated toward work. Despite this, I felt the need to engage my mind differently and picked up reading as a hobby. It's incredibly relaxing, and much of what I share with you comes from what I've read. But it's no longer just work for me; reading and writing have become a refreshing escape and growing experience."

Be Open to Humor

Embrace moments of joy and laughter. Laughter is not only a delight but also a boon to your well-being. It can alleviate stress, soothe tense muscles, and flood your brain with feel-good hormones. Consider indulging in some stand-up comedy, spending time with friends, or seeking out humorous clips on social media. Whatever it takes, ensure you carve out moments to smile and laugh. Remember, amidst life's hustle, you deserve these pockets of joy.

"I remember spending time with my best friends or family when I was a kid, and we'd end up in those fits of laughter, lying on the floor and laughing uncontrollably. I recently experienced this joyous feeling again during the workshop I attended. Just be kids again, never forget who you are, and treasure your inner child."

Follow a Healthy Lifestyle

Engaging in physical exercise can help alleviate feelings of anxiety and stress for you. When you choose cardio routines like cycling, jogging, or running, you're allowing your heart to work at its best, circulating oxygen-rich blood throughout your body. These activities don't just lift your spirits; they also strengthen your muscles. By maintaining a consistent sleep pattern, you give yourself the gift of proper rest and the joy of waking up refreshed every morning. Embracing a healthier lifestyle is not just beneficial; it's a compassionate act towards yourself, paving the way for a more fulfilling life.

"Many face the same challenge I once did. Believe me, the desire to unwind at home is strong after a long day at work. However, that's not always the best approach. Instead of settling in immediately, consider walking with your dog or hitting the gym. Shaking up your routine can be invigorating. Once I began, it became an enjoyable activity, a way to meet new people and develop personally. So, I encourage you to get moving!"

Be Compassionate to Self and Others

Your strength and resilience are incredible tools that enable you to uncover deep wells of compassion. Remember to uphold your emotional equilibrium and steer through feelings with grace. Grant yourself the same compassion you offer others, and never forget how deserving you are of love and kindness. When change doesn't manifest instantly, refrain from being overly critical of yourself. Realize that every challenge or misstep you encounter is a hidden lesson waiting to be embraced. Approach each moment with a heart full of hope and unwavering mental fortitude.

RELATABLE STORIES

- "I realized that fear and anxiety stem from the change I'm encountering and the brain's adaptation to that change, and also to the uncertainties that lay ahead. Rather than believing that these negative feelings are something 'wrong' in my life, I've realized that this is part of the human condition: change, uncertainty, and concern. I've learned to embrace these feelings, and that has brought me a tremendous sense of comfort," (PunctualPoetry, 2021).
- "When we look at nature, we can see that everything is always in a state of transition; there is no true stagnation in life. People often think that always sensing you're in a state of transition means there's unhealthy instability, but the transition and moving forward are actually signs that you're progressing. Waiting for the next thing to 'stabilize' isn't the right way to view these moments because you'll never actually begin to thrive," (edgar_vpacos, 2021).
- "I like to live my life as though before I came to earth, I agreed to everything that would happen to me as a way to learn and help others learn. This means that despite all of the uncertainty, it's all happening for my greater good. Life happens for me, not to me. It helps me be

more accepting and grateful for every experience, knowing that I've already said yes to them," (Mrs. Michael Moore, 2021).

Anxiety, fear, and worry can be challenging to navigate, but your journey through them is incredibly valuable. Throughout this chapter, you've been introduced to strategies, attitudes, and mindsets that can help you embrace and manage those challenging emotions. Adopting a resilient and optimistic mentality can empower you to cultivate a sense of inner peace. Building and maintaining strong relationships and seeking professional guidance when needed are essential steps in your pursuit of enhanced emotional well-being. Now, together, let's move forward, ready to dismantle **negative thought patterns** and find confidence in your newfound ability to rise above challenging emotions and foster a more harmonious life.

3

BREAKING NEGATIVE THOUGHT PATTERNS

> *People look for retreats for themselves, in the country, by the coast, or in the hills. There is nowhere that a person can find a more peaceful and trouble-free retreat than in his/her own mind... So, constantly give yourself this retreat, and renew yourself.*
>
> — MARCUS AURELIUS

Negative thought patterns are often driven by fear and uncertainty. To combat these detrimental thoughts, you need to learn how to replace them with more uplifting and empowering ones. When you become aware of these negative thoughts and recognize the damaging effects of such thinking, you'll be better positioned to reframe and reshape them, offering yourself compassion and shifting your perspective.

It's not uncommon for individuals to fall into negative thought patterns, especially when grappling with mental health issues like depression, anxiety, or low self-esteem. These irrational thinking patterns can adversely influence your emotions and actions. Confronting and transforming these patterns isn't a one-time task; it demands consistent effort and commitment. Seeking guidance from a support group or a mental health professional can be invaluable in challenging and redirecting these thought patterns.

There isn't a single, clear-cut cause for negative thoughts. Yet, many experts believe that a significant portion of our thoughts tends to be negative and repetitive. When these thoughts become overwhelming, they distort your perception, leading to unrealistic views of yourself and your surroundings.

Allowing negative thoughts to dominate can pave the way for self-sabotaging behaviors. In this chapter, the aim is to guide you through effective strategies to address and diminish the mental challenges exacerbated by these negative patterns, which might have been amplified by experiences like the pandemic or other life adversities. Together, we'll pinpoint these thoughts, nurture a resilient mindset, and better equip you for any future hurdles with understanding and compassion.

This is the second **'B' in the B-BRAVE framework.**

Recognizing Negative Thought Patterns

The first step you need to take in overcoming negative thought patterns is to become familiar with them. Just as with any challenging experiences or emotions, you need to muster the courage to face them head-on. Once you're able to address these negative patterns with understanding, you'll find a pathway to making peace with them.

Everyone can get ensnared in the downward spiral of negative thoughts; you're not alone in this. It's especially common when faced with difficult situations. Here are some insights and strategies to help you navigate and combat these challenging thought patterns.

Introduction to Negative Thoughts or Hungry Ghosts

Occasional negative thoughts may be fleeting and might dissipate over time. However, if any of these thoughts go unaddressed, they can intensify, leading to irrational thinking and behaviors.

- As you journey through self-awareness, consider reflecting on the following:
- Do you sometimes replay unpleasant moments or experiences, wishing you could change their outcomes?
- Do uncertainties about the future ever lead you to envision the bleakest scenarios?
- Do you find yourself seeking constant validation or approval from specific people to feel complete?
- When things don't unfold as planned, do you find it easy to place blame on yourself or others?

It's completely natural if you resonate with some or all of these questions. Such patterns can lead your mind down a path of heightened worry. Remember, transforming these thoughts into positive ones is a journey, not a destination. It may require patience, practice, and kindness toward yourself to cultivate the mental strength and determination for change. Always be gentle with yourself as you navigate this path.

"For me, it took years of introspection, self-awareness, and countless self-help books to overcome these negative thought patterns. However, when the pandemic hit, it felt as if a switch had been flipped. Did I feel as though all my progress had been undone? Absolutely. It was a poignant reminder of how our environments can deeply influence our thoughts and emotions."

DEFINITION OF NEGATIVE THOUGHTS OR HUNGRY GHOSTS

According to Hawkley (2013), negative thoughts are perceptions, expectations, and attributions tinted with unsettling emotions. Negative thoughts in your mind can resemble hungry ghosts, ceaselessly feeding off your positive emotions. They seldom find satisfaction, and if left unchecked, these patterns may expand. Such thoughts tend to loop, heightening your susceptibility to depressive symptoms and intensifying emotional disturbances.

It's essential to recognize that persistent negative thinking can overshadow any rays of optimism in your life, stealing away moments of joy and hindering your ***journey toward*** a fulfilling existence. Remember, acknowledging and allowing these feelings is the first step to healing and growth.

What Causes Negative Thought Patterns?

 "I learned that the roots of negative thoughts may start physically, psychologically, or spiritually. Always check in with yourself."

— PETER LAST

It's important to remember that there isn't just one root cause for these feelings; they can stem from a multitude of factors. Your negative thinking patterns might differ based on your unique experiences, triggers, surroundings, and the support you've had. Sometimes, negative thoughts can originate from the subconscious, reacting to specific situations, like when you feel emotions such as jealousy, anger, or self-doubt. It's okay.

The state of your subconscious mind can influence those spontaneous thoughts that come into your conscious awareness. Remember, you're not alone in this, and understanding is the first step toward healing.

"Some of my negative thought patterns existed from childhood traumas I experienced."

Negative Thinking vs. Negative Self-Talk

Negative thinking and self-deprecating inner conversations can restrict your ability to see the bright side of life. Negative thinking becomes a pattern, causing you to expect the worst outcomes, which in turn can influence your actions. Engaging in negative self-talk means you're often being too harsh on yourself, magnifying your mistakes and missteps.

Everyone has that inner critic, but consistently succumbing to such self-talk can feel like you're constantly punishing yourself, potentially eroding your trust in your own abilities. Think of this inner voice as an overly critical companion, one who sometimes doesn't know when to stop. For instance, if you earned a C on a science test, this voice might convince you that you'll never excel in that subject. Such internal dialogues can sap your confidence, making it challenging to initiate positive shifts in your life. Remember, treating yourself with kindness and compassion is the first step towards breaking this cycle.

"I want you to understand that this journey requires dedication and effort, especially if you've found yourself deeply ensnared in negative patterns. I personally felt as if I was trapped, having to carve a way out. But with the guiding light of the Ho'Oponopono prayer, I found a path to healing and hope."

TYPES OF NEGATIVE THOUGHTS

There are various types of negative thoughts, each involving different ways of thinking. Below are a few examples of negative thoughts you may need to reflect on.

All-or-Nothing Thinking

When faced with a challenge, we might find ourselves thinking *nothing goes as planned* or that little failures are the absolute end. These thoughts are thinking in black and white, often going into downfall when experiencing setbacks.

Overgeneralization

Overgeneralization is a pattern of negative thinking where one expects that one bad event will lead to an endless chain of misfortunes.

Mental Filter

When you linger on a particular negative thought, it can cast a shadow over your other thoughts and perceptions. Just as a single drop of ink can cloud clear water, this negative thinking can make it challenging for you to see the bright side. Remember, it's natural to feel this way at times, and by acknowledging these feelings, you're already taking the first step toward finding clarity and healing.

Disqualifying the Positive

Similar to the mental filter, when you focus on a certain negative element, you sometimes refuse to accept positive experiences. Often, these positives are filtered out so they **"don't count,"** and you end up rejecting the positive experiences in your life.

"This is basic manifesting 101."

Jumping to Conclusions

This kind of thinking has you leaping to a negative interpretation of an event, even when there's no clear evidence that such an outcome will occur.

"What I refer to is the confused hamster mind."

Mind Reading

When you meet someone new, you might assume they're forming negative opinions about you. You're letting your perception of their impressions overshadow your self-view, even if those assumptions may not reflect reality.

"Are you grasping the power of the mind?"

The Fortune-Teller Error

You feel convinced that whatever bad things you think will eventually be true. As if you're a fortune-teller, you feel like your predictions are established facts, and they will happen sooner or later. This can be, for most, the downward spiral of life; **_perceptions can become a reality._**

Magnification (Catastrophizing) or Minimization

It is healthy to recognize our flaws and weaknesses, but if we take these imperfections too seriously, it can be harmful. We might be dismissive or ignorant of our own strengths and other positive qualities.

"That's where I've learned to love my mistakes; they are lessons in disguise."

Emotional Reasoning

You make quick judgments based on your negative emotions, letting your negativity define your reality of what's happening. In some cases, you might be doubting your intellectual capabilities in certain areas of your life; therefore, it must be true. This habit will lead you to make decisions based on your emotions alone rather than trying to be reasonable or objective.

Rational Thinking:

It refers to logical or reasoned thought processes based on objective evidence. Rational thinking involves objectively considering all available facts and information and making decisions based on this evidence, free from bias or emotional influences.

Irrational Thinking:

It is not grounded in objective reality or logic. It's often influenced by emotions, misconceptions, or biases, leading to beliefs or decisions that might not make logical sense when examined closely. Personal beliefs, emotions, or unfounded assumptions can sway irrational thinking.

"Should" Statements

Instead of seeking resolution or expressing remorse when you make a mistake, do you often veer towards self-deprecation or defeat, telling yourself that you deserve or ought to feel bad?

"Don't beat yourself up, you're only human and being the best, you can be!"

Characteristics of Negative Thinking

Negative thoughts can sneak up on you in various forms, often catching you off-guard and sometimes skewing your perception during crucial moments. These thoughts might even be so compelling that you momentarily question your core beliefs. It's crucial to realize the potential damage of this negative self-talk.

Research has shown that dwelling on past mistakes and engaging in self-blame can amplify feelings of helplessness, hopelessness, and depression. By frequently immersing yourself in these negative narratives, you might inadvertently add to your stress levels, veering away from reality and hampering your progress toward your goals.

This mindset can also dim your vibrancy, affecting your relationships and clouding your perception of others. It can eat away at your confidence, making you feel less equipped to handle challenges and inhibiting you from seizing opportunities. Remember, it's perfectly natural to experience these feelings at times. However, know that you possess the strength to grow, learn, and shift towards a more positive mindset, ensuring you maintain both mental energy and focus on your personal growth.

INCREASED RISK OF OBSESSIVE-COMPULSIVE DISORDER (OCD)

OCD is characterized by repeated thoughts, often becoming an obsession. These thoughts are typically related to "perfect" conditions. When negative thoughts become a habit, they may become an obsession, potentially intruding on daily life.

Cognitive Distortion: When Negative Thinking Forms a Larger Pattern

A cognitive distortion is fueled by continuous negative thinking, exaggerating our "thinking errors" and biased judgment. Cognitive distortion acts as an internal mental filter that merely exacerbates our misery, making us feel bad about ourselves. It's an inaccurate and irrational way of thinking and is automatic and often subconscious, usually occurring without us even noticing. Consulting with a professional therapist or a hypnotherapist is recommended to challenge this thinking.

Habits that Lead to Cognitive Distortion

There are thinking habits that might increase your risk of cognitive distortions. When you fall into these patterns regularly, they can influence your daily life and challenge your ability to think rationally. You might feel apprehensive about attending social events, burdened by insecurities and self-doubt.

While it's beneficial to make thoughtful decisions, when these decisions are consumed by negative self-talk, it begins to impact your mental well-being. Overthinking can be exhausting, pulling you into a whirlwind of imagined scenarios and making you feel the need to control every situation.

Such thinking can be counterproductive when the expectations you've carefully crafted don't align with reality. Then there's the trap of rumination: constantly revisiting painful memories or past mistakes. Reflecting on past experiences can be a path to growth, but when it's overshadowed by self-criticism, it can take a toll on your mental health. And then, there's the weight of cynical hostility, which can strain your relationships and make you see others through a lens of distrust or suspicion. Remember, understanding these patterns is the first step to navigating them with kindness and compassion toward yourself.

Solutions to Overcome Negative Thoughts

Nurturing your mental well-being is crucial for combating negative thoughts. Just as one trains their muscles for strength, cultivating a habit of processing information positively can significantly bolster your mental health. Remember, it's about training your mind to perceive situations in a healthier, more constructive light.

While acknowledging challenges is essential, addressing them with a mindset that promotes growth can be transformative.

Always keep in mind that setbacks are often stepping stones in disguise. Embrace the belief that regardless of the obstacles you face, you possess the resilience and capability to address them.

Despite moments of sadness, anger, or regret, there's always an opportunity for you to rise and shine anew. To counteract negative thinking and create emotional balance:

- Prioritize physical well-being through regular exercise, consistent sleep, and a balanced diet. They're not just beneficial for your body but also elevate your mood and energy.
- Foster deep connections. Engage in heart-to-heart talks with loved ones, letting their comfort and understanding support you through turbulent times.
- Don't shy away from seeking professional help. Therapists can equip you with strategies to tackle negative self-talk and address core issues.
- On the spiritual front, consider aromatherapy, proven by research like that of Hung et al. (2023), to reduce stress and fatigue. Connect with a higher power, be it through prayers, rituals, or meditation, offering solace and a renewed sense of purpose.
- Engage with spiritual communities. Building connections with like-minded souls can fortify your emotional well-being, providing a shared journey of understanding and growth.

ACTIONABLE WAYS TO TURN NEGATIVE THINKING INTO POSITIVE THINKING

Stay anchored in the present moment. When ensnared by dark ruminations, allow yourself to be enveloped by the world outside. Pause, breathe, and immerse in the vastness of the sky or the brilliance of the sun. Such gentle pauses can draw you away from the turmoil and center you in the soothing embrace of the now.

Embrace journaling, a sanctuary for your deepest feelings and a catalyst for self-awareness. Should overwhelming thoughts arise, find a quiet space, and audibly declare, "Stop!" This simple affirmation can disrupt the cascade of negativity, guiding you back to clarity. And if ever you're harsh with yourself, draft a list celebrating your strengths and qualities.

Reframe your thoughts, asking: "Would I ever say this to someone I care about?" Realize that you deserve the same kindness and tenderness you'd offer to a cherished friend. Every step you take is a testament to your journey toward self-compassion and understanding.

RELATABLE STORIES

- "Be aware of your mind when you are thinking negative thoughts. When you catch it, take a deep breath and acknowledge the negative thoughts. Let it go and pay attention to what you were doing," (Jamsto, 2018).
- "Train your brain. The Buddhists believe the brain is a

muscle that can be worked. Focus on the thoughts you don't want or the things you don't want to say. Repeat to yourself (in your head) 100 times to not think or to not say that. Every time it comes up, another 100 times," (BeerMania, 2018).

- "The first thing that you should know is that you should be aware of yourself, and if you find yourself having these kinds of thoughts, don't punish yourself. Investigate how to develop some self-compassion because that's where it all starts. I used to punish myself even for the pettiest things, and it does you literally no good. Because you can't think of solutions from that position, so be nice to yourself first," (Topper, 2018).

Banishing negative thought patterns is a journey that requires dedication and practicing perspective shifts. By recognizing these unhealthy thinking habits, we can perceive the world differently, see challenges as a way for growth, and develop a healthier relationship between our mind and body.

SHIFTING PERSPECTIVES ON FEAR, WORRY, AND ANXIETY

Shifting perspectives is like discovering a new way to view a room you've always known. You're already familiar with its contents, but suddenly, you're seeing it in a whole new light. The same holds true for your feelings of fear, worry, and anxiety: you know these emotions intimately, yet now we'll attempt to view them from a fresh perspective.

It's natural to become entangled in traditional definitions of fear, worry, and anxiety, thinking of them as adversaries that harm you mentally and physically. Yet, there's a gentle way to perceive them that's less intimidating: by focusing on the broader landscape of your life.

In this section, you'll uncover compassionate approaches to ***navigating anxiety***, offering you a renewed understanding and path forward.

Shifting Your Perspective on Fear

Everything that challenges you is an opportunity for growth. Remember when you were young and took that tumble from your bike, scraping your knee? Though it hurt, over time, those wounds healed. And if you fell again, the sting was less sharp, and you knew how to cope.

It's like exercising; when you lift weights, you might feel that ache from the minor tears in your muscles, but this is how you grow stronger. Just as your body adapts and becomes resilient, so does your mind.

To fortify your mental muscles, sometimes you need to step beyond what's familiar. Embracing the unfamiliar can be daunting, but confronting those fears signifies growth. There may be hurdles along the way, but trust that the journey is enriching. Embrace the discomfort, for in it, you'll find the strength to be at ease with the unease.

How to Begin Overcoming Your Fears

You might start by identifying activities or situations that stir up feelings of unease or apprehension. Maybe cooking feels daunting due to worries about making errors, letting others down, or wasting food. Recognizing and documenting this fear, alongside the potential repercussions of sidestepping the challenge, offers clarity. For instance, avoiding cooking might mean more money spent on take-outs or veering from healthy eating goals. But remember, when you gently confront these fears and embrace moments that might challenge your confidence, you unlock a deeper self-awareness. Just think about the common fear of public speaking. By taking small steps, like sharing insights in intimate groups or joining discussions, you'll find that each experience boosts your confidence. With every challenge faced, your comfort zone broadens, and you pave the way for both personal and professional growth. Embrace the journey, for it's in the stretch beyond our fears where true growth lies.

Manage Worry by Perspective Shifting

Worries often anchor you in a single, unyielding place. When you dwell on your anxieties, you might overlook the vast tapestry of your life. Yet, you're right here, living this very moment. Why let future uncertainties cloud your present? Dwelling on them can deplete your mental energy, leaving you focusing on aspects beyond your control and feeling stuck. Here are some gentle suggestions to help shift your perspective and ease those worries.

Remember Your Mortality

Sometimes your worries can become so consuming that you lose sight of how fleeting and precious life truly is. While many of us hope to reach old age, everyone's journey is unique. However, pausing to reflect on those anxieties and then zooming out to a broader perspective can be healing. For instance, will that one challenging day at work yesterday truly overshadow the beauty of your entire life? Certainly not; your life holds far more value than a singular rough day.

Make a Timeline

Reflect on the journey you've taken over the past decade. Recognize the vast difference between who you were then and who you've become today. While it's easy to dwell on recent challenges, pause and ask yourself: How many of those concerns still weigh on your heart? Often, taking a moment to put today's worries in perspective can be a soothing balm, breaking the cycle of endless stress. And when the weight feels too heavy, lift your gaze to the heavens. The vast sky, with its twinkling stars and gentle winds, serves as a humbling reminder of life's transient nature and the incredible gift of simply being here and experiencing it all.

Understanding the Brain Helps to Put Things into Context

Your brain, beyond its incredible complexity, holds the keys to understanding your emotions and reactions to stress. By delving into how parts like the amygdala (your emotional epicenter) and the prefrontal cortex (which tries to keep those emotions in check) function, you unveil the mysteries of your own reactions.

When faced with challenges, your amygdala might amplify those stressful emotions, causing you to focus more on potential threats than on solutions. Studies, like the one by Pizzagalli in 2011, even found that those with depression tend to have heightened activity in these emotional zones.

By recognizing and understanding these inner workings, you can nurture a deeper connection with yourself, empowering you to separate from the stress and find healing, especially if anxiety has been a shadow in your life.

Navigating away from negative thought patterns is a journey that calls for your unwavering commitment and a willingness to see things anew. By identifying these limiting beliefs, you're unlocking the power to view challenges as stepping stones and foster a harmonious bond between your mind and body. Embracing practices like mindfulness, treating yourself with gentle compassion, or even seeking professional guidance can pave the way for uplifting and affirming thoughts. Remember, true change is a gradual dance, so be patient and tender with yourself. As this chapter concludes, ask yourself: *"Do these thoughts truly align with my highest or better self?"* As we turn the page, you'll delve deeper into reshaping those **core beliefs** that shape your world.

4

REVISING CORE BELIEFS

> *Authenticity is an alignment between your beliefs, your desires, and your choices in the world. Desires that are in alignment with core beliefs generate powerful actions. Like a wave that draws from the depths of the ocean, actions connected to your authentic self are more likely to manifest your intentions.*
>
> — DAVID SIMON

Identifying Core Beliefs and Their Influence

In the wake of the pandemic, you might find yourself harboring newfound fears or suspicions. Perhaps you've grown wary of others, questioned the narratives surrounding the virus, or felt frustrated by government policies. These feelings could subtly shape your core beliefs, nudging you towards a mindset of mistrust or the idea that life has turned irrevocably unfair.

Recognizing and reassessing these deep-rooted beliefs is vital. I urge you to gently reflect upon and challenge any limiting or negative convictions you hold. With an open heart and a willingness to change, you can adopt beliefs that not only empower you but also enhance your connections with others.

Embracing this transformative mindset is the **'R' in the B-BRAVE framework**, a pivotal step in forging a path of understanding and resilience.

What Are Core Beliefs?

At the core of your understanding of yourself and the world around you lie core beliefs. These powerful principles shape how you view yourself, others, and the environment you navigate daily. Often, you might not even be conscious of these beliefs, yet they operate like a set of unspoken "rules" governing your interactions and perceptions.

While some of these beliefs uplift and empower you, many, unfortunately, might hold you back, painting a picture of a world that feels rigid and unchanging. Imagine harboring a belief that, despite all evidence of your accomplishments, your subconscious still whispers that you're not quite good enough or any negative pattern held. Or perhaps these deep-seated convictions unknowingly lead you to form biases influenced by past experiences or societal norms.

It's essential to recognize and gently challenge these beliefs, for they shape your interactions and feelings, both toward yourself and others. Remember, by understanding these core beliefs, you open a path to transform your perceptions and the richness of your relationships, experiences, and ultimate healing growth.

Examples of Core Beliefs

Not all of your core beliefs are rooted in negativity; many can be uplifting or neutral. The journey is about nurturing these positive beliefs within yourself. Here, you'll find some examples to gently guide you, offering a starting point to recognize and embrace your core beliefs.

Beliefs About Goodness

These are beliefs that some people are good or bad based on certain behaviors or traits. This is also applicable to other people around them or their surrounding environment. Examples of negative core beliefs about goodness include:

- "I am a bad person, and that's just who I am."
- "Other people are not trustworthy—I will always face betrayal."
- "Everyone is inherently evil."

However, there are instances where someone can have good faith in themselves and in the world around them. Their core beliefs may include more positive ones, such as:

- "I am a kind person, and I will try to always do good."
- "Everyone is worthy of my kindness."
- "Everyone is capable of doing good things."

Beliefs About Likability

These beliefs are linked with how much some people feel they are likable or unlikable. Common negative core beliefs include:

- "I am unlovable, and nobody will love me."
- "I don't have friends, so I must be a freak."
- "Nobody wants to hang out with me because I'm not likable."

These beliefs can be so deeply ingrained that some people end up growing unfriendly and always suspecting everyone of thinking badly of them. So, let's see how positive core beliefs can be empowering in contrast.

- "I know people will need time to see the value in another person."
- "I have friends; that means I'm likable enough."
- "I'm a funny person and people like my jokes."

Beliefs About the World

It's easy to perceive the world as negative with all the tragedy that has happened. The pandemic only exacerbates these beliefs. Common negative perceptions about the world include:

- "The world is a dangerous place."
- "The world is corrupt."
- "The world is unjust."

How we see the world mirrors how we act for our environment. If we believe that the world is inherently a bad place, we place little to no respect for nature and may worsen the conditions of the world itself. So, let's see how positive and optimistic beliefs may change our behavior:

- "The world is a wonderful place."
- "The world is full of magical things."
- "The world is the perfect place to be alive."

Beliefs About Competence

Doubting abilities or competence may start from core beliefs. Negative examples of beliefs about competence include:

- "Failing means I'm bad at it."
- "I'm not skillful like everyone else."
- "I'm not a smart person."

There may be some things that hold us back from trying again—be it from failure or frustration—but believing in ourselves incapable of improvement and change is not going to help. Let's see how positive examples can change perceptions.

- "I will succeed if I put my mind to it."
- "I have my own unique sets of skills and interests."
- "I'm learning to be smarter every day."

WHERE DO CORE BELIEFS COME FROM?

Many elements from your early years have molded your core beliefs. These beliefs might spring from the embrace of your family, the lessons learned at home or school, and the myriad experiences that marked your youth. As you've journeyed through life, seeking clarity and purpose, you've held onto certain beliefs to guide your path. Yet, it's essential to remember that some of these beliefs, formed so early, might not always reflect the full truth of who you are and the world around you.

Think about it: there might have been a time when you believed the rain was the sky's way of shedding tears, a belief that might've stayed with you longer than you'd admit. These core beliefs, whether true or not, play a pivotal role in defining who you are, not as innate truths but as lessons and patterns you have absorbed over time.

Adversities like childhood bullying, harsh words from parents, or other heart-wrenching moments might have sowed seeds of negative beliefs in your mind. Sometimes, the lessons and beliefs from your younger days can lead you to assume everyone sees the world just as you do. But remember, your unique journey doesn't mirror everyone else's.

There's profound strength in seeking guidance. Collaborating with a therapist can illuminate those shadowed beliefs, helping you reshape them into affirmations that resonate with your true self, fostering growth and understanding.

CORE BELIEFS: HOW THEY INFLUENCE YOU AND WHAT TO DO ABOUT IT

Core beliefs affect everything we do. An inaccurate view of reality can sometimes lead to cognitive distortions, believing something completely false that may be harmful to us or the people around us. If I absolutely believe that I am a person of no value, I may never believe in other people's compliments, thinking they are always lying and constantly looking down on me. This, in turn, can kill self-esteem overall and make us believe we are not worthy of love. This can happen to children, especially those coming from broken marriages, who lived, learned, and grew from it.

So, what to do about harmful core beliefs? Do you hide from them or face them?

 "Don't be a slave to stupid rules."

— DR. JORDAN B. PETERSON

Identifying Core Beliefs

Recognizing your core beliefs can be a subtle journey, but let's walk through some nurturing steps to illuminate them. Begin by tuning into those spontaneous thoughts that often whisper unnoticed, and embrace your feelings, whether uplifting or challenging.

They might be mirrors reflecting your deepest beliefs. Consider journaling a few times a week, especially during emotionally charged moments. Jotting down those raw feelings after a disagreement or during moments of introspection can be illuminating. After you've penned your thoughts, revisit them.

Do you often find yourself taking undue blame? Dive deeper and ask yourself why. Is there an underlying belief that your voice is less significant? Through this gentle introspection, you can unwrap layers of beliefs, understanding yourself more profoundly and compassionately.

Considering Evidence

When you find yourself wrestling with your core beliefs, taking a moment to truly reflect on the evidence behind them can be enlightening. Gently and compassionately assess how valid and reliable that evidence really is. Remember, by objectively understanding what fuels your beliefs, you're granting yourself the opportunity to grow and find deeper clarity in your journey.

Here are examples of how evidence can support both positive and negative core beliefs:

Positive core belief: "I am capable and deserving of success."

Evidence supporting this belief:

1. Past achievements: I have accomplished various goals and received recognition for my abilities.
2. Skills and talents: I possess specific skills and talents that others have recognized and appreciated.
3. Positive feedback: I consistently receive positive feedback from peers, mentors, and supervisors regarding my capabilities and performance.

Negative core belief: "I am unworthy of love and affection."

Evidence supporting this belief:

1. Past rejection: I have experienced instances of rejection or abandonment in relationships, reinforcing the belief that I am unworthy of love.
2. Negative self-perception: I tend to focus on my perceived flaws and shortcomings, leading me to believe I do not deserve love or affection.
3. Limited positive experiences: I have had few positive experiences in relationships or receiving love and affection, reinforcing the belief of unworthiness.

Remember, your core beliefs, intricate as they may be, deserve thoughtful reflection. It's essential for you to examine the evidence behind them with a discerning eye. By courageously challenging and reshaping those deep-seated beliefs, you embark on a transformative journey toward personal growth and cultivating a healthier mindset. Embrace this journey with kindness to yourself, understanding that this exploration is a profound act of self-care and love.

Core Beliefs Play a Role in Addiction

Your core beliefs shape so much of your world, influencing your mental health and the connections you make with others. If these beliefs lean towards the negative, feeling unsupported or seeing oneself as fundamentally flawed can become all-consuming.

Such beliefs might push you towards unhealthy habits or relationships, possibly leading you to find solace in substances like drugs or alcohol. Believing that you're inherently bad or incapable of change weighs heavily on the heart, fostering feelings of depression, self-doubt, and even self-loathing.

In an attempt to escape these overpowering emotions and quiet the harsh self-talk, you might find yourself drawn to temporary reliefs, which can, over time, evolve into an addiction. This path can further cement the belief that you're undeserving of love and assistance.

What's more, the societal stigma around addiction can make it even harder for you to reach out. But remember, understanding this connection is the first step to healing and finding your way back to a compassionate view of yourself.

You Can Identify and Challenge Core Beliefs

Your core beliefs, though deeply rooted, can be redefined with dedication and effort. The beauty of your mind lies in its adaptability; it can evolve, just as your behaviors and habits can. If you ever feel entrapped by these beliefs, consider seeking the guidance of a professional therapist. Through CBT, they can assist you in recognizing the distressing parts of your life, perhaps those shaped by past trauma or challenging relationships. They'll guide you in identifying the beliefs and behaviors that are tied to your pain, help challenge those distorted beliefs, and aid you in crafting healthier, more constructive ways of thinking. Remember, it's a journey, and with each session, you're one step closer to understanding and empowering your true self. You deserve to be free from the shackles of negative beliefs and to embrace a brighter, more positive future.

RELATABLE STORIES

- "What are beliefs? For me, it was what someone told me to be true. It's literally a perception of the world. Someone else who didn't grow up like I did has a completely different perception of life. It's not real. And why hold on to them? What purpose does it serve to have a negative outlook on the world? Stop holding on to these beliefs that aren't serving you. You'll be surprised at what's holding you back," (Public_Past694, 2021).

- "For those that are not aware of their negative beliefs, one way to do this is to write about positive affirmations of what you want in your life that isn't currently your experience. Just work on a couple at a time, writing each like ten times a session, and as you are writing them down, listen and pay attention to the inner critic, 'Yeah, but...' and on another page, write those reasons down. Those are your core negative beliefs to change," (Anonymous, 2021).
- "Practice watching your thoughts. Part of what defines a 'core belief' is that many other beliefs and habitual thoughts are connected to it or built upon it. If you're serious about re-examining your core beliefs, you will find that you have to re-examine a lot of other ideas too. Treat those thoughts with the same open-mindedness that has caused you to question the core belief and overwrite the pathways with the same patient repetition of more balanced, chosen thoughts," (G Scrap, 2022).

Changing core beliefs can be tough since it's a belief that has been planted deep inside our subconscious. However, through thought reframing and professional therapy, if needed, challenging negative core beliefs is doable.

RESTRUCTURING AND ADOPTING EMPOWERING CORE BELIEFS

Embarking on the path of restructuring and embracing empowering core beliefs can be a transformative journey for you. By confronting those negative beliefs and reshaping them into positive, uplifting ones, you have the potential to unlock profound personal growth and enhance your well-being. Remember, every step you take towards understanding and reshaping your beliefs is a step towards a more fulfilled you.

Here are two examples of empowering core beliefs I have adopted:

1. Old belief: "I am destined to fail at everything I attempt."

Empowering core belief: "I am capable of learning and growing from every experience, and success is within my reach."

By reshaping that belief, you've begun to see setbacks and failures not as dead ends but as invaluable stepping stones for growth and insight. When challenges arise, you now face them with unyielding resilience and a hopeful heart. Understand that every stumble, every misstep, can be the very thing, that propels you toward greater success. Remember, it's not about never falling, but about rising each time you fall, stronger and wiser than before.

2. Old belief: "I am not worthy of love and affection."

Empowering core belief: "I deserve love and can build healthy, fulfilling relationships."

By challenging those lingering doubts, you've come to a beautiful realization: you are worthy of love and nurturing relationships. This transformative belief has paved the way for more robust self-worth and deeper, more genuine connections with those around you. Through dedication and introspection, you're reshaping those foundational beliefs, gravitating towards empowering viewpoints that brighten your world. Understandably, this evolution requires time and patience. Yet, every step you take on this path of self-discovery and growth promises rewards that are truly immeasurable.

What Are False and Self-Limiting Beliefs?

You might have felt it before, that nagging voice inside you that whispers, "You're not enough," or "You'll never find love." These self-limiting beliefs, often negative and rooted in untruths, may hold you back, making you feel trapped in a version of yourself that isn't reflective of your full potential. Throughout this section, let's embark on a journey together to unpack and transform these limiting beliefs into empowering thoughts that can propel you forward.

False and self-limiting beliefs are those assumptions you may hold about yourself or the world that aren't necessarily true and can hinder your growth and success. Consider the belief, "I'm not good enough." This thought might make you feel inherently inadequate, dampening your self-confidence and possibly stopping you from chasing opportunities. Yet, if you look closely, you'll find unique strengths within you that are capable of crafting successes in various aspects of your life. Or take the belief, "I'll never find love." Such a belief can paint a bleak picture of your future relationships. But remember, love is within reach for everyone, and by nurturing self-love and personal growth, you pave the way for meaningful connections.

Recognizing and challenging these beliefs is vital. By transitioning to a mindset that champions your potential, you welcome a world brimming with opportunities and new horizons.

So, where do these self-limiting beliefs originate? Let's delve into a framework introduced by Milton Rokeach in 1968, known as the hierarchical system of beliefs. This system categorizes beliefs into five levels based on their significance.

Your most basic beliefs, those which you've never thought to question, like family ties or the language you speak, fall into Type A. These are the beliefs you've likely accepted without thought. Then there are Type B beliefs—those core beliefs about yourself and others that shape your identity. These foundational beliefs often form early in life.

Type C beliefs arise from authority figures you might have looked up to – perhaps a parent, a teacher, or a mentor. Over time, you might have placed enormous trust in their guidance, which inadvertently shaped some of your self-limiting beliefs. Type D beliefs, or peripheral beliefs, stem from aligning with specific systems or ideologies. For instance, if you identify with a particular expert's opinion, you might adopt their views, even if they might not be entirely accurate.

Lastly, Type E beliefs, as Rokeach described, are more fluid and may change based on experiences, like developing new tastes or preferences.

Now, considering false or self-limiting beliefs, Rokeach particularly pointed to Type B and Type C beliefs as the culprits. When you let others influence your perceptions and feelings, you might find yourself bound by deeply rooted beliefs they've instilled. Recognizing these origins can be the first step to breaking free and redefining your narrative with compassion and empowerment.

Therapeutic Options to Combat Self-Limiting Beliefs

There are a few therapeutic options for you to challenge self-limiting beliefs. The therapeutic options we will discuss here include Rational Emotive Behavior Therapy, Cognitive Restructuring, and Schema Therapy.

Rational Emotive Behavior Therapy (REBT)

REBT offers a beacon of understanding and self-awareness, illuminating the dark corners of your mind where negative or irrational thought patterns might reside. Imagine going through life held back by chains of self-limiting beliefs. REBT is the key to breaking those chains and setting yourself free. Its structural approach is especially helpful for anyone wrestling with behaviors affected by limiting beliefs, guiding them toward clarity and empowerment.

Imagine you've poured your energy into an essay and, with a mix of pride and trepidation, handed it over for grading. The next day, your inbox pings with an email from the professor with detailed feedback attached. Your heart sinks even before you read the first word. Without delving into the details, feelings of worthlessness and incompetency start to bubble up; your irrational thoughts say you've let your professor down and didn't meet their standards. But if you took a moment and read through the feedback, you'd realize there were constructive critiques and, nestled at the end, a sincere compliment on your good work. Yet, those initial negative emotions had already cast their shadow, making you doubt your capabilities.

Let's decode this using the ABC model of REBT:

1. A stands for the "Activating event," the spark that lights the flame of doubt. Here, it's that lengthy feedback you received.
2. B represents the irrational "Beliefs" that rush in afterward. In your case, it's the mistaken idea that your work was subpar and that you aren't up to the mark.
3. C signifies the "Consequences," the emotional fallout from harboring these misconceptions. This can lead you to feel dejected and question your competence.

Understanding these triggers is the first step. Once you've laid them bare, you can confront them, using mindfulness to halt those first negative thoughts in their tracks. Cognitive restructuring becomes your tool, helping you swap out those irrational thoughts with balanced, fairer ones. Then, you can employ relaxation techniques to soothe and reclaim your emotional equilibrium.

REBT is not just a method; it's a journey to rediscover and champion yourself. Embrace it, and watch as you transform challenges into opportunities for growth.

Cognitive Restructuring

Cognitive restructuring offers you a compassionate lens through which you can interpret, reflect upon, and understand the events and emotions surrounding your life. Rooted in the principles of Cognitive Behavioral Therapy (CBT), this technique is best explored alongside a trained therapist, ensuring you traverse these mental pathways safely and constructively.

Imagine attending a session where your therapist guides you through "Event Questioning," a method specifically designed to gently challenge and reshape your thought patterns. You'll be encouraged to share a recent stressful experience and express how it made you feel. As you share, the therapist may gently interject with thought-provoking questions designed to illuminate areas of potentially irrational thinking.

They might ask:

- "What concrete evidence supports this negative thought you're feeling?"
- "Are these thoughts stemming more from an emotional place or from clear evidence?"
- "Could there be underlying assumptions influencing how you feel right now?"

Some common examples to positively reframe your defeating beliefs include:

- Failure is an opportunity to learn. When I see failure as the absolute end, it's a harmful belief to keep me from trying again. To challenge this, I will replace this defeating belief; I can see that failure is a learning experience and a chance to improve myself.
- Look at the bigger picture. When faced with a problem, I tend to see situations from a very limited perspective. Next time, when I'm caught up in a stressful moment, I try to "zoom out" of my current situation and see the world as if I were a bird flying high in the sky. The "bigger picture" can help me stay balanced in my position.
- Look at it as if you were a different person. When trying to see an issue through another person's perspective, it might instill new ideas, insights, or information that we wouldn't notice.

- Things could be worse. This positive reframe allows you to practice gratitude and be grateful for what you have. It's important to remind yourself that your life is enough, and you could be in a worse situation.

To put this into context, consider an example where you've received feedback on an essay. After reading the professor's comments, the therapist would gently encourage you to evaluate if there was clear evidence suggesting incompetence. Was there specific feedback implying you weren't suited for the course? Or was it possible that these thoughts sprouted more from assumptions or purely emotional reactions?

Through cognitive restructuring, you're given a compassionate space to dissect and understand your thoughts. The journey aids you in separating emotions from evidence, fostering a more balanced and positive perspective on the challenges you face.

Schema Therapy

Schema therapy is a compassionate approach designed to help you address long-standing beliefs, often formed in childhood or adolescence. These deeply ingrained beliefs, or schemas, aren't just fleeting thoughts or momentary cognitive distortions; they've taken root over the course of your life. They've become a part of your internal narrative, guiding your actions, reactions, and perceptions of the world around you.

Schemas can be tough to alter. They've weathered time and life experiences, making them persistent companions in your journey.

The therapy required to address them tends to be long-term, giving you ample space and time to understand, confront, and eventually change these core beliefs. Reflecting on our earlier discussion about Type B and C beliefs, it's these deeply entrenched perceptions about identity, self-worth, and self-image that often give rise to these limiting and sometimes detrimental beliefs.

Some familiar schemas that might resonate with you include:

- Subjugation: a feeling that you should always yield to others' desires or judgments.
- Punitiveness: an internalized idea that you deserve punishment, even for mistakes that aren't your own.
- Failure: a pervasive sense that you're destined to fail, no matter how hard you try or how worthy your efforts are.

Let's consider a relatable example to bring this closer to home. Imagine you've written an essay, and a voice inside you immediately whispers it's not good enough. That voice might be echoing a failure schema. Think back. Can you recall an instance in your early years, perhaps a stern teacher who criticized your work without reason? Such experiences can sow the seeds of these schemas, but remember, with understanding and compassionate therapy, they can be confronted and changed.

How to Change Your Limiting Beliefs for More Success

Often, you might not realize where your limiting beliefs come from, and this unawareness can hinder your well-being. These beliefs tend to nestle deep within your subconscious, influencing your emotions and how you perceive the world.

To tackle these beliefs, it's crucial to become more in tune with your subconscious. Start by analyzing your environment and pinpointing triggers that might awaken these beliefs. Imagine those moments when you feel isolated and overwhelmed—what past events might be driving these emotions? Maybe as a child, you felt overlooked or unsupported by those who were meant to care for you, leading to feelings that persist into adulthood. Such experiences could shape a belief that you neither deserve help nor should extend it to others, constraining your potential.

The journey to change begins by questioning these deep-rooted beliefs. Understand that some of these beliefs have been handed down for generations. Embrace new perspectives and actively seek ways to break free from these outdated molds. Remember, you hold the reins of your life, actions, and happiness. Don't allow external factors to control your decisions. You're at the helm of your destiny, steering towards what truly resonates with your core values and dreams. Empower yourself to design the life you wish for, choosing a mindset that not only combats those limiting beliefs but also welcomes a world of joy and possibilities.

REFRAMING DEFEATING BELIEFS AND LANGUAGE

There are a few ways we can practice reframing defeating beliefs into more empowering ones. These methods require us to reframe a few languages or phrases to be more encouraging to our thoughts.

Empowering Language

Here are a few examples to replace discouraging language with empowering phrases:

- Replace **I have to…** with **I choose to; I want to…**
- Replace **I should have…** with **next time I can…**
- Replace **I'm just; I'm only…** with **I am…**
- Replace **I try to…** with **I commit to; I aim to…**

Reframing Through Coaching

Seek a professional therapist to help you bring awareness to disempowering language you may be using. A therapist can offer new perspectives and give you a chance to look for opportunities if you were to change your thoughts, moving them into a more powerful perspective.

Disempowering Languages	Empowering Questions from a Coach
"I have no choice; I have to/must/can't do this."	What if you knew you had a choice?
"I'm not like everyone else; I'm too lazy/incompetent/stupid for this thing."	What happens if you were to let go of those labels?
"It's all my fault; I screwed up."	What if there was no one to blame?

Work with your coach or therapist to bring your negative thinking into light, challenging your self-limiting beliefs to be more optimistic.

Empowering Beliefs to Live By

Here, I want to share a few examples of empowering beliefs that you can say to yourself.

　1. I believe in myself.

You are the only person who can make a change for yourself. Believe in your abilities and handle everything in life with an open heart and an open mind.

　2. I know how to heal.

There are moments of grief and moments of happiness. In times of sorrow, you always know that there will be an opportunity for you to rise again.

3. I choose what's right for me.

Other people's expectations of you aren't what truly matters. Learn to manage your own expectations first and take action based on what you believe is right rather than getting swayed by others' opinions of you.

4. I know my strengths.

You'll focus on your strengths and hone them rather than getting caught up in your weaknesses. You won't let your imperfections define you or weigh you down.

5. I'm open to changes and new possibilities.

You are always open to fresh opportunities, eager to embrace new knowledge. Give yourself the freedom to experience both the highs and lows, for they'll shape your growth. You can forge new friendships, dive into a novel hobby, and let new experiences enrich your life.

Transforming deeply held beliefs can feel daunting, as they're rooted deep within your subconscious. Yet, with tools like thought reframing and even professional therapy, when necessary, you have the power to challenge and shift these limiting beliefs. All it requires is your heartfelt commitment to embrace change. Embracing mindfulness can be your salve, healing the mental scars left by these negative core beliefs. Journey with me into the next chapter, where we'll delve deeper into **adopting mindfulness.**

HEY THERE, ENTHUSED READER, BEFORE JUMPING INTO THE NEXT CHAPTER!

First, thank you for diving into "Courageous New Dawn: Mastering Your Mindset - Mastering Your Mindset Understanding Anxiety - Learning to Thrive with Fear in an Ever-Changing World!" It means the world to us that you've chosen to embark on this transformative journey.

Let me ask you this: have you ever wished you had known about a life-changing book or resource sooner? That's where your review can make a monumental difference, in someone else's life.

Thank you in advance for your contribution. You're awesome!

Happy reviewing!

Common Sense Factor

5

ADOPTING MINDFULNESS

> *The still waters of a lake reflect the beauty around it. When the mind is still, the beauty of the self is reflected.*
>
> — VANDA SCARAVELLI

Mindfulness might have its roots in Buddhist practices but embracing it doesn't require any religious affiliation. Perhaps you've come across mentions of mindfulness in articles, books, or other self-improvement discussions. At its core, mindfulness invites you to be fully present, to immerse yourself in the current moment. It's about truly feeling your thoughts, body sensations, and surroundings without getting entangled in past regrets or future worries. Imagine the solace in that—living in the now, especially in these tumultuous times.

Adopting mindfulness can directly counteract any COVID-related fear and anxiety.

In the aftermath of the pandemic, practicing mindfulness can be your sanctuary against the tides of fear and anxiety. When you welcome mindfulness into your life, you're nurturing an awareness that helps you steer through change and unpredictability with grace. It's a transformative process, turning waves of anxiety into a calm sea of clarity and deliberate action.

Incorporating mindfulness not only dissipates the shadows of pandemic-induced concerns but also attunes you to your innermost feelings and responses. It fosters a deep understanding and compassion—for yourself and for those around you. This essence of being present, to truly understand and empathize, represents the **'A' in the B-BRAVE framework.**

Introduction to Mindfulness and Its Benefits

You might often wake up with thoughts already racing, plotting out your day filled with work and household duties. Amid this whirlwind, it's all too easy to feel disconnected from the world and, perhaps more poignantly, from yourself. Lost in the maze of past regrets or wishes for a different now, you may miss the beauty of the present moment.

Mindfulness offers a gentle embrace, urging you to center your focus on the here and now, welcoming it without judgment. This practice is not just about grounding; it's a gateway to diminished stress and amplified joy. As we journey through this section, you'll uncover methods to heighten your awareness of the present and truly grasp the transformative magic of mindfulness.

Practices for Improving Emotional and Physical Well-Being

There's a world of mindfulness practices awaiting your discovery. Among the most transformative are mindfulness-based stress reduction (MBSR) and mindfulness-based cognitive therapy (MBCT). Imagine embracing the teachings of Jon Kabat-Zinn through MBSR, guiding you through daily activities to anchor you firmly in the present moment. Then there's MBCT, a harmonious blend of cognitive behavioral therapy with mindfulness, often chosen to support those with depression, guiding them away from potential relapse.

While these techniques can offer solace to those facing mental challenges, consider this: there's compelling evidence suggesting that embracing mindfulness not only aids in healing but can also fortify your mind against future struggles. Picture yourself nurturing a sanctuary within, enhancing not just your mental well-being but also your overall physical health. Your journey to wellness awaits.

What Are the Benefits of Mindfulness?

You might be surprised by the wealth of scientific studies revealing the profound effects of mindfulness on well-being. Embracing mindfulness can be a transformative tool for managing chronic pain, alleviating anxiety, and panic disorders, mitigating depressive symptoms, overcoming addiction, and addressing various other challenges. Whatever your age or walk of life, these mindfulness techniques are waiting to offer you peace and harmony. Let's journey together as we uncover the myriad of ways mindfulness can enrich your life.

Navigating a world that sometimes feels overwhelming, especially in the aftermath of a global pandemic, you're not alone in seeking solace. Have you felt the weight of fear and anxiety, those constant stressors? By embracing mindfulness, you'll find a pathway to respond more effectively to life's challenges. When you practice mindfulness, it becomes a tool, allowing you to process and cope with stress in healthier ways.

We've all had those challenging days at work, moments of negativity that seem hard to shake off. Mindfulness offers you a sanctuary, a way to process and allow these feelings rather than push them away. Research has even shown that mindfulness-based cognitive therapy can provide lasting relief for those battling depressive symptoms. But the benefits don't stop at your emotional well-being. As you cultivate mindfulness, you're also investing in your physical health. Studies, such as one by Black (2016), have indicated that a consistent mindfulness practice can bolster the immune system. And that restless sleep you might be experiencing? Techniques like MBSR can help enhance sleep quality.

For those grappling with chronic illnesses, either personally or watching loved ones suffer, the emotional toll can be immense. While mindfulness might not be a cure, it certainly brings a sense of relief, managing symptoms, and promoting relaxation. Even caregivers and family members can benefit from reducing anxiety and depressive feelings. And if you or someone you know struggles with addictions know that mindfulness offers a beacon of hope, helping diminish cravings and prevent relapses. Remember, in this journey toward well-being, mindfulness can be your trusted companion.

How Does Mindfulness Work?

Mindfulness invites you to embrace your negative emotions or experiences rather than pushing them away. Many mindfulness approaches are intertwined with other healing practices, like psychotherapy, meditation, and cognitive behavioral therapy. Recognizing the profound influence of these mindfulness techniques demonstrates the profound depth of healing and understanding they can offer you. Embrace this journey, for it's a compassionate path to true self-awareness and inner peace.

Mindfulness Techniques

Mindfulness, in its many forms, offers a gateway to serenity, focus, and a deep-rooted connection to the present. It's about grounding yourself amidst the whirlwind of life's challenges, anchoring your thoughts, and acknowledging the world around you. As you embark on this journey, let's explore some techniques tailored just for you to guide you through the myriad landscapes of your mind.

Basic Mindfulness Meditation: Find a serene corner and settle down. As you take a deep, nourishing breath, turn your attention to the sensations coursing through your body. Thoughts, like fleeting shadows, might dance at the edges of your consciousness. Instead of resisting, simply let them come and go, granting them passage without letting them steer your emotions.

Body Sensations: You might become aware of subtle tingles, itches, or other sensations. Instead of reacting, embrace this moment of acute awareness. Traverse your consciousness from the crown of your head down to the tips of your toes, embracing every sensation and heartbeat.

Sensory Connection: The world around you teems with stimuli. Sounds might whisper to you, or lights might flicker at the edge of your vision. Perhaps you could enhance your focus by enveloping yourself in gentle meditation music. Identify each stimulus, holding it in your mind's eye for a fleeting second and then gracefully letting it go.

Emotional Recognition: Emotions, both uplifting and challenging, are part of your tapestry. Instead of shying away, name each emotion as it surfaces. It could be a gentle wave of nostalgia or a storm of jealousy. Recognize its presence, breathe out, and then release it into the ether.

Craving Urge Surfing: If you're grappling with powerful urges or cravings, remember they, too, are transient. Witness the pull they exert on you, the way they ripple across your being. Instead of succumbing, send out a silent wish, a beacon of hope, willing these cravings to recede. Ground yourself in the present, reminding yourself of the impermanence of these urges and the strength that lies within your heart, mind, and spirit.

Mindfulness Meditation and Other You

Meditation is a wonderful doorway to weave mindfulness into your daily life. Whether you choose to journey alone or seek the companionship of a mindfulness instructor or meditation group, the shared energy of others can bolster your commitment and invigorate your practice.

Starting on your own is simpler than it might seem. In the beginning, all you need to do is tune into your breath. Give yourself the gift of just five minutes a day, and let that foundation grow. As you delve into this practice, aim to sharpen your concentration, attune to your inner thoughts and feelings, and embrace the present. It's natural to have your thoughts drift to yesterday's memories or tomorrow's plans, but gently guide yourself back. Embrace each sensation, each emotion, without judgment. At times, it may feel challenging or even a tad overwhelming, but with patience and dedication, you'll find that it becomes more intuitive. Trust in the process; it's a journey that promises to deepen your self-awareness and comfort in your own skin.

Moreover, meditation teaches the art of acceptance, urging you to embrace whatever surfaces in the present moment. Treat yourself with kindness and compassion, recognizing that the wandering mind is part of the human experience. If you find yourself veering off into self-doubt or daydreams, lovingly bring your focus back to the now. Remember, every breath offers a fresh start. And outside of your formal meditation sessions, seize opportunities to practice mindfulness in everyday activities. For instance, when eating, savor every bite, immersing yourself fully in the experience, letting each morsel nourish both your body and soul. It's a journey of gratitude and presence.

MINDFULNESS EXERCISES

I'd be delighted to guide you through some mindfulness exercises that you can embrace within the comfort of your home. These gentle practices are handpicked with love and care, hoping they bring solace and presence to your moments. Remember, this journey is all about you. Dive in and allow these practices to illuminate your path to inner peace.

Basic Mindfulness Meditation

- Find a comfortable position and stick with it. Sit on a chair or cross-legged on the floor with your back straight.
- Focus on your breathing. Feel the sensations as the air flows through your nose or your mouth, or your chest rising and falling with every breath you take.
- Once you have gained concentration, begin to widen your focus. Become aware of the sensations, sounds, ideas, emotions, and thoughts.
- Embrace these thoughts and emotions without judging. If your mind starts to wander on a specific memory, return your concentration to breathing, listen intently, then begin expanding your awareness again.

Learning to Stay in the Present

- Start by bringing attention to sensations in your body.
- Breathe in through your nose, allow the air to flow through your body, and let your abdomen expand fully.
- Breathe out through your mouth slowly.
- Notice the sensations of each inhalation and exhalation.
- Proceed with your current task slowly with full concentration.
- Engage within your senses fully. Notice each touch and each sound, and savor everything with your senses.
- If you notice that your mind has wandered from your current task, bring back your attention to the task you are doing right now, and focus on the sensations of the current moment. Focus on your breathing as a quick return.

Invest in Yourself

The journey of mindfulness meditation might not yield immediate results. Understand that it requires consistent dedication and discovering the approaches that resonate with your unique needs. With persistence, the transformative effects will begin to unfold. Many find that the true benefits of meditation become palpable about 20 minutes into their session, emphasizing the importance of patience. Cherish and invest time in yourself. Begin your meditation practice gently, perhaps with just five minutes, and gradually extend your sessions. It's warmly recommended to immerse yourself in 45 minutes of meditation at least six days a week. Remember, this journey is as much about self-love as it is about self-discovery.

CULTIVATING PRESENT-MOMENT AWARENESS

The end of the pandemic, the beginning of the war in Ukraine, ongoing global political tensions and changes, and the alleged climate crisis fueled by flash fires worldwide have brought a fresh set of concerns to your doorstep. *How will the future shape up? Will things ever revert to what they once were? Are you with me? It's crazy out there!* And the lives lost, the moments missed —could there have been a different path? Such worries, built upon each passing moment, can seem endless, leaving you little reprieve. Amidst these concerns, there's the present: a beautiful, fleeting moment that often goes unnoticed. Recognizing and cherishing this present becomes an essential gift.

Dwelling on bygone times or incessantly wondering about the future can amplify feelings of despair, anxiety, and unease, robbing you of the joy the present moment holds and lowering your vibration. In this section, I'll walk you through cultivating an awareness rooted in the here and now. Realize that life is unfolding right this moment. It's said that lingering in the past can bring sorrow, while constantly looking ahead stirs anxiety. Remember, your imagination shapes the future you envision. The present, however, is genuine, immediate, and truly a treasure to be cherished.

What Is the Present Moment?

The present moment is a fleeting bridge between your past and your future, a delicate balance where life manifests in its most genuine form. It's the sensation of your chosen medium beneath your fingers, the gentle cadence of your thoughts as they shape your reality. The present is where you reside, where you learn and interact. It's that fleeting second you grasp and reflect upon, a continuous now that neither dwells in what was nor rushes to what will be. Your unique journey involves discerning the values and beliefs that serve you right now, deciding what to embrace as truth or set aside as mere distractions, and contemplating whether these align with your deeper aspirations. This is your present moment; what does it mean for you?

Your past, interlaced with inner child trauma memories and experiences, can either constrain or bolster your growth. When you tune into the rhythms of your thoughts, you might find moments of unease, triggering reactions that might not serve your current situation. Dwelling on bygone times or nervously awaiting what's next can be a disservice, considering the past is set, and the future is unwritten. Recognizing and healing from old wounds is an ongoing journey. Remember, the only true moment you have, the one where life genuinely unfolds, is now.

How do Mindfulness and Present-Moment Awareness Relate?

Mindfulness and present-moment awareness speak directly to you, entwining seamlessly with the core essence of compassion. When you embrace compassion, you not only acknowledge the suffering around you but also feel a deep-seated urge to ease it. Likewise, when you practice mindfulness, you invite a kind, non-judgmental gaze upon your own experiences, which is essentially an act of self-compassion. By anchoring your attention to the here and now accepting life's ebb and flow without judgment, you're nurturing a kinder and more compassionate relationship with yourself.

This compassionate approach to mindfulness magnifies your connection to the present, radiating outwards from you. As you grow more in tune with your emotions, thoughts, and sensations moment by moment, you also unlock a deeper understanding of those around you. You become finely attuned to the intricate tapestry of human emotions and interactions, making you more capable of extending that same compassion outward. In this way, by immersing yourself in mindfulness and being truly present, you pave the way for richer, more empathetic connections with your inner self and the vast world surrounding you.

The Benefits of Present-Moment Awareness

- increased quality of life
- greater sensations of pleasure
- improved mental clarity
- enhanced ability to empathize with others
- decreased anxiety and other negative moods
- better emotional regulation
- better immune system
- enhanced concentration

Achieving present-moment awareness requires you to clear your mind of any worries and truly immerse yourself in the now. When you attain mental clarity, your productivity and concentration flourish. Being truly present allows you to handle daily tasks with ease as you dedicate yourself to one thing at a time.

Giving your undivided attention to a singular task can dramatically enhance your creativity and productivity. While some might champion the benefits of multitasking, it's often a deceptive efficiency booster. It might appear more effective to some, but for many, it leads to divided attention and reduced quality of work.

Have you ever felt that juggling several tasks at once drains you faster? Instead of achieving more, distractions pull you in different directions. The constant switch between tasks can leave you feeling scattered as your brain tirelessly jumps from one endeavor to the next. Remember, it's okay to focus on one thing and to give yourself the grace to be present in each moment.

"Navigating the deluge of information about the pandemic and other global concerns, I often felt overwhelmed and uncertain. My mind was a whirlwind, constantly questioning which sources were reliable and beneficial for me. Questions like, "Should I trust the science behind the vaccine?" and "Is it possible for a vaccine to be developed so rapidly and still be safe?" became significant sources of anxiety in my life.

"Many of you might have had different concerns related to the situation, stirring up anxiety. Thoughts such as wanting to find the best way to shield your loved ones from the virus or feelings of devaluation when labeled 'non-essential' in a society you've

contributed to for years. It's natural to harbor resentment or anger towards the virus in such situations. However, these emotional responses can affect your vibrational energy, potentially clouding your judgment and leaving you feeling detached or numb to the ongoing circumstances."

Scientific Research on Present-Moment Awareness

You might find it intriguing to know that there's a study showcasing how mindfulness meditation can be a beacon of relief for those grappling with trauma. Imagine the relief and empowerment one might feel, knowing that there's a way to better handle those overwhelming emotions linked to past distressing events. The fascinating part? This study employed MRI scans, delving deep into the brain's reactions. Among the participants, some were expert meditators with two decades of practice under their belt.

Have you ever lain awake at night, thoughts racing, yearning for a night of deep, uninterrupted sleep? You're not alone. But here's a glimmer of hope: certain research suggests that by simply being present, by grounding oneself in the here and now, not only can the quality of your sleep improve, but it might also offer solace to those wrestling with sleep disorders. Beyond just sleep, embracing the present moment has been linked to reduced stress and an alleviated sense of discomfort among those enduring chronic illnesses.

But there's more. Dive a bit deeper, and you'll encounter findings that illuminate the potential of mindfulness practices in treating

PTSD. For those haunted by past traumatic events, cultivating a practice of being truly present can offer a nurturing space—a buffer, if you will—between painful memories and the promise of the present moment. Imagine the solace and freedom that comes with that separation, allowing healing to take center stage.

HOW TO CULTIVATE PRESENT-MOMENT AWARENESS

In today's fast-paced world, it's easy to lose yourself in reflections of the past or dreams of the future. But have you ever paused to truly feel the magic of the present moment? Taking the time to be fully present can transform your experiences, offering you profound moments of clarity and joy. Imagine allowing yourself the grace to be truly present, connecting deeper with yourself and the world around you.

How can you harness the beauty of the present moment? Start with a gentle body scan. As you lie back in the serene corpse pose, allow your mind to traverse through each part of your body, feeling every sensation. Ground yourself; press your feet firmly to the earth, embrace nature, or simply hug yourself, reminding yourself of the present. Embrace the tranquility of mindful walking, feeling every step, every sensation. Listen with all your heart, absorbing every word in conversations, leading to richer connections. Gift yourself moments amidst nature, feeling its soothing touch and reconnecting with its wonders. Lastly, delve into the world of art as "Jim Carrey" did during the pandemic. Whether you create or simply appreciate, art has the power to pull you into the now, making you more attuned to every nuance.

Allow these practices to be your gateway to the present, your sanctuary amidst this chaos of a world gone mad.

How to Stay in Control

With a deep connection to the present moment, you can achieve greater mastery over yourself. When your thoughts wander to the past or future, they can quickly veer off course, pulling you away from the present. Therefore, for the best harmony of mind and body, it's essential for you to remain anchored in the here and now. Remember, true control comes from embracing and being fully present in this very moment, with kindness and understanding towards yourself.

Here, I want to share a few tips to help you stay in control.

- Trust in your existence
- See yourself as a whole person—enough and thriving
- Always favor cooperation over competition
- See other people as equals, treat them with respect and common decency
- Heal yourself regularly, exercise all, whether it's mental, physical, or spiritual
- Realize that the only reality is the present moment
- Believe in your growth, see yourself as a being of constant evolution

Integrating Mindfulness into Daily Life

Practicing mindfulness can be done everywhere, not only in individual sessions. Besides focusing on one task at a time, I encourage you to integrate mindfulness activities into your daily life. Here are a few examples of simple mindfulness activities that you can practice throughout the day.

Mindfulness Activities You Can Practice Throughout the Day

In a world that often feels like it's in overdrive, it's essential to find moments of stillness and mindfulness. Your journey to a more balanced life starts with the simple act of gratitude. Begin each day by focusing on one positive thing in your present moment. Allow that warmth to envelop you, serving as a gentle reminder of the blessings that surround you. When emotions bubble up, pay attention to your heart's rhythm. Is it racing with anxiety? Slow down and anchor yourself with a deep breath. Remember, your breath is a powerful tool in recalibrating your emotional compass; inhale the good you want to see in the world and exhale the negative.

As you navigate through your day, let your five senses be your guide. Relish in the world around you: the colors, sounds, textures, and scents. This immersive experience can be especially transformative during meals. Practice mindful eating; let each bite be an exploration, savoring the unique flavors and textures. In your interactions, listen to understand, not just respond. Your words carry weight, so choose them with intention. Amid the day's demands, don't forget to pause, even if just for a moment.

These intentional breaks can serve as a sanctuary, grounding you and reminding you of the beauty in the present moment and being your true self.

RELATABLE STORIES

- "To me, being mindful is to not over-identify with our ego. It allows for a shift in perspective at times when the ego keeps us stuck. My interpretation is that there is a self, which is the totality of our being. However, this being is without a static essence. It can change and grow and is largely ungraspable. On the other hand, the ego tries to materialize itself into the static and absolute center of our being, the focal point of control. This is what mindfulness counteracts. It allows us to let go of whatever dogmatic interpretations we hold of ourselves," (ullemaiseenstoephoer, 2022).
- "Mindfulness is an observer. You shouldn't be passing judgment. Openly accept everything, that includes your thoughts, feelings, and sensations that actively pop into your mind. These are just simply distractions to your concentration that will subside as your mind quiets over time. Remember, don't get frustrated when you lose focus often. These are all stepping stones to develop your mindfulness," (findurapiotr, 2018).
- "Mindfulness will bring lots of emotions and feelings forward. Try not to resist your feelings. Embrace it. Don't think about how in the future you may or may not be alone. Settle into what's going on right now. Accept

it. Love it. I promise, if you work with it, you will no longer feel lonely when you are alone! It's a really amazing feeling," (sb11345, 2019).

Mastering mindfulness might feel like an overwhelming task, but with dedicated practice and unwavering commitment, you have the power to heighten your awareness of the present moment and refine your responses. It's essential to remember that there's no universal blueprint for mindfulness; finding what resonates with you might take time, just as it does for many others. Embracing mindfulness demands focus, consistent effort, and a heart open to change and transformation. A pivotal step in this journey? Addressing procrastination head-on. Stay with me, as the upcoming chapter will lovingly guide you through compassionate strategies to **vanquish procrastination** and embrace the present.

6

VANQUISHING PROCRASTINATION

 The momentum of continuous action fuels motivation, while procrastination kills motivation.

— STEVE PAVLINA

We've all faced the pull of procrastination, haven't we? It can cloud our productivity, pulling us into a whirlwind of guilt and shame. When you find yourself in its grasp, it can feel like a relentless cycle, difficult to escape, yet draining your momentum each day. And let's be honest: with the uncertainties you've navigated since the pandemic, it might seem like procrastination has found an even more tenacious foothold in your life.

Now more than ever, it's essential to kindle that spark of motivation and action to rise above these procrastinating tendencies. You can forge a proactive mindset by understanding the roots of your delays and hesitations. This won't just quell the rising tide of anxiety but will also light the way to renewed productivity and resilience as we enter a post-pandemic world.

We delay and defer for many reasons, but by mapping out a clear path, dividing our tasks into bite-sized pieces, and setting realistic targets, you can conquer that urge to postpone. And trust me, nurturing motivation and discipline is your best ally in crafting a proactive approach toward your aspirations.

Addressing and managing these feelings is pivotal to dissipating fear and anxiety. You have the tools within you to rise above procrastination, fueling your drive and boosting your productivity. This proactive approach is the **'V' in the B-BRAVE framework**, guiding you toward a brighter, more productive future.

Why Do You Procrastinate?

Sometimes, you might find yourself putting things off, and it's natural to feel this way. Procrastination often emerges from emotions you might be intimately familiar with, a fear of making a mistake, a feeling that a task might be tedious, or even worries about not living up to expectations. Occasionally, the sheer complexity or volume of tasks can feel overwhelming, nudging you into delay. It's genuinely compassionate to delve deep into understanding the emotions that drive you to procrastinate. Could it be that this behavior has a purpose in your life? Let's explore this together, gently and without judgment.

UNDERSTANDING THE PSYCHOLOGY OF PROCRASTINATION

You might understand procrastination as a tendency to delay or push off tasks until the very last moment or even beyond a deadline. But consider this: procrastination isn't always your enemy. Effective time management means prioritizing what's crucial and setting aside what's not as pressing. Actual procrastination strikes when you commit to a task and then neglect it or give it up for no valid reason.

Even while fully aware of the repercussions of postponing your responsibilities, you might still succumb to procrastination. Have you ever felt that, ironically, overcoming procrastination seems even more daunting than just tackling the task at hand? It's a curious mix of self-deception and a tussle with self-discipline.

Many studies on procrastination reveal that it's especially prevalent in academic and professional environments, making it a frequent companion for students and office workers. While work-related stress, looming deadlines, and decision-making dilemmas often push you toward this habit, it's essential to understand that the roots of procrastination go deeper. It's not just about work fatigue or burnout; your mental and emotional state plays a significant role. With empathy and understanding, let's delve into the core reasons why you might procrastinate, the repercussions it brings, and the distinct profiles of procrastinators out there.

What Are the Psychological Roots of Procrastination?

Your mental state plays a pivotal role when it comes to procrastination. You might sometimes feel a lack of confidence, anxiety, or perhaps struggle with time management. Maybe, on some days, the motivation wanes, or the task at hand feels too ambiguous even to begin. Psychologists have discovered that negative emotions, in particular, play a significant role in this.

Procrastination often intertwines with rumination—those moments when you're caught up in spirals of negative thoughts or self-talk. Remember, it's completely human to feel this way; understanding these feelings is the first step toward addressing them.

Does Procrastination Serve any Purpose?

Procrastination might initially feel like a comforting blanket, shielding you from fear and anxiety. It's understandable; sometimes, it's a way to guard your mental well-being, ego protection. However, when it becomes a frequent visitor, it can cultivate a damaging pattern of self-doubt, making it even harder for you to face challenging tasks head-on.

Isn't it true that, as perfectionists, you might sometimes use procrastination as armor? It's a way to defend against the daunting shadows of potential failure, judgment, and self-criticism. Avoiding tasks that seem unpleasant is a natural instinct. And while immersing yourself in more delightful activities (*"substance abuse"*) can feel like a solace in the moment, remember that there might be repercussions. Know that in these feelings, you can find a way forward through understanding and self-compassion.

"When negative thoughts arrive, I ask, is it a rational or irrational thought? Does it serve my higher purpose? Being present is critical in understanding and allowing these thoughts."

The Consequences of Procrastination

Procrastination can have far-reaching effects, encompassing emotional, physical, and practical realms. If you frequently delay tasks, the quality of your work might suffer. Over time, this could foster a pattern of negative self-talk, which may increase the risk of mental challenges like depression and diminished self-worth. This avoidance behavior can make it even more challenging for you to map out your future, as you might start to doubt your capacity to set goals and maintain motivation.

Moreover, if procrastination seeps into matters of physical health, such as putting off exercise, delaying medical checkups, or neglecting healthy eating and sleep routines, the consequences could be detrimental. Remember, every step you take today can shape a healthier tomorrow. Embrace each moment and know you have the strength to move beyond procrastination. Let's journey together toward productivity and well-being.

Causes of Procrastination

You probably recall when you promised to clean your apartment or reorganize the garage. Maybe you even gave yourself two full weeks to accomplish it, only to find that it remained untouched. You might often tell yourself it's just not the "right time" because you aren't "feeling it" or lack motivation. It's easy to underestimate how long a task will take, giving you a comforting illusion that there's ample time ahead. Yet, often, you find that the task goes undone until, perhaps, it's too late.

One of the sneaky culprits behind procrastination is the belief that you must be in the perfect mood or mindset to tackle a task. But if you're always waiting for that ideal moment to strike before cleaning the apartment or diving into any project, you might discover that moment rarely arrives. The longer you delay something, the easier it becomes to put it off repeatedly until it slips off the radar entirely.

Let's explore a few other factors holding you back from diving into tasks. Remember, understanding the root causes of procrastination is the first step toward overcoming it. We're all on this journey together and seeking guidance and self-reflection along the way is okay.

Navigating the academic world isn't always a smooth journey. If you find yourself frequently delaying assignments. Studies suggest that a staggering 80% to 95% of college students grapple with procrastination, particularly when faced with challenging coursework. It's easy to overestimate the time at hand or underestimate the complexity of a task. Sometimes, you might believe you need to be in the "right mood" to start, or you could be fearing criticism. And isn't it often tempting to prioritize instant gratification over a demanding project, like watching a favorite show?

Procrastination isn't just about pushing things off; it can also hint at deeper underlying issues. Depression, for instance, might rob you of the motivation to act. Obsessive-Compulsive Disorder (OCD) might amplify fears of making mistakes, and Attention Deficit/Hyperactivity Disorder (ADHD) can scatter your focus, especially when a task doesn't captivate your interest. If you're wrestling with these feelings, there's no shame in seeking help. Remember, understanding the root of procrastination is the first step toward overcoming it. Embrace self-awareness, seek understanding, and know that every day offers a fresh opportunity to move forward.

Overcoming Procrastination Through Effective Planning

Navigating the challenges of the post-pandemic world, have you, too, found procrastination creeping into your daily life? Maybe the shifting routines, the comfort of home, or the uncertainty of the future has made it easier to say, "I'll do it tomorrow." Yet, as we mold ourselves to fit the contours of this new normal, it becomes essential to rekindle motivation and tackle procrastination head-on.

You might wonder: Why the delay? Is it laziness or procrastination? The two are different. Procrastination is choosing a lesser task over a more important one, while laziness is indifference to action. Remember when you kept postponing a significant undertaking, filling your hours with inconsequential activities, and waiting for the elusive "right mood?" Acknowledging this behavior is the first step. Dive into the reasons behind your procrastination. Perhaps fear of a task's difficulty or anticipation of discomfort holds you back. Starting small can make a mountain seem like a molehill.

It's vital to remember that habits, especially procrastination, aren't unraveled overnight. Tackling it requires kindness to oneself and strategic planning. Organize with a to-do list, break down larger tasks, recognize when you're most productive, set tangible deadlines, and employ the wonders of technology like time-management apps such as Trello or Notion. And if you stumble? Forgive yourself. Each day is a fresh slate, and each task completed, no matter how small, is a step forward. Motivate yourself with rewards and reframe your internal dialogue to one of empowerment. Choose action, not because it's demanded, but because it's a step towards your goals. Remember, with your journey, determination, and compassion for oneself, the chains of procrastination can be broken.

"Writing this book has impacted my procrastination and triggered anxiety, and so the limiting beliefs arise; maybe the book is unnecessary, or the big one is my friends and family will think I'm nuts for sharing my thoughts in a book and letting others know my issues. When the student is ready, the teacher arrives, and from my healing, it's important to share as it may trigger and help another heal. You see, we are indeed not alone. I'm still here and so are you, so let's celebrate our courage to come this far."

Reverse the Procrastination Triggers

In your journey towards productivity, you might recognize specific "procrastination triggers" that push tasks into the "I'll do it later" category. Does this sound familiar?

- Finding a task tedious or unrewarding?
- Feeling overwhelmed by how unstructured or ambiguous it is?
- Believing it's too tricky or lacks personal meaning?

When these triggers arise, they often overpower the logical part of your brain, making emotions reign supreme. Suddenly, you're scrolling through social media or chatting with friends instead of tackling that important task.

Yet, remember, there's hope. There are strategies to guide your logical brain back into the driver's seat. Firstly, work within your resistance. Everyone has limits; if an hour feels overwhelming, start with a manageable 20 or 30 minutes. Commit to it. Secondly, just make a start—any start. Diving into the task, even a tiny part of it, can often break the mental barrier. Before you know it, you'll find that things aren't as daunting as they first appeared. Also, occasionally remind yourself of the costs of procrastination. What are the ripple effects of pushing that task aside? Will it impact your family, future stress levels, or even your standing? Remember, kids are very impressionable at a young age; create a game for you and your children to overcome this procrastination you are experiencing and have fun.

Lastly, electronic devices can be a siren call of distraction in our increasingly digital world. Consider giving yourself tech breaks. Silence notifications or even stash your phone away while working. You create a sacred space for focus and productivity by muting those digital disruptions. Embrace these techniques with kindness and patience; they are your allies against procrastination's pull.

BUILDING MOTIVATION AND DISCIPLINE TO TAKE ACTION

Throughout your journey, you've undoubtedly encountered numerous obstacles and distractions that have held you back or led you astray from your goals. Unresolved inner child traumas leading to feelings of self-doubt, procrastination, external pressures, and unexpected setbacks might have dimmed your drive at times.

With its swift and unexpected challenges, the COVID pandemic has likely reshaped your perspective on motivation and discipline. The abrupt shift from traditional workspaces and learning environments to remote settings has blurred the lines between personal and professional realms, possibly making it harder for you to concentrate and maintain motivation.

But remember, the first step to reignite that inner spark is to reconnect with what genuinely drives and inspires you. You can uncover your true passions, values, and purpose by fostering motivation and discipline. This cultivated discipline can reinforce your commitment to your chosen path and bolster your resilience against life's adversities. These are vital tools to help you refocus on your aspirations and maintain a strong sense of self and work ethic amidst these rapidly changing times.

In the following section, you'll find strategies tailored to help you foster the right mindset, enabling you to build habits that support your motivation and discipline. Embrace these methods in your daily routine and equip yourself to navigate the uncertainties of our post-pandemic world with renewed confidence and clarity.

What Is Self-Discipline and Its Importance?

Self-discipline is the power to manage impulses and emotions, centering attention on the task at hand. Decision-making and staying true to long-term goals can be a challenge, especially when distractions or hurdles appear. Isn't it tough sometimes? The allure of immediate rewards can be tempting, and it's entirely natural for the brain to crave them. For a balanced and fulfilling life, it's essential to weave self-discipline into every facet, from personal habits to work commitments and even the care of your mental and physical health. It's about setting transparent goals, nurturing routines, and mastering time. Remember, every step you take towards self-discipline is a stride toward your most authentic self. Embracing self-discipline doesn't require you to be unbending or to confine yourself too tightly. Instead, it's about cultivating habits that resonate with your core values and aspirations. It's giving yourself the grace to make mindful decisions that propel you toward personal growth, ensuring you feel supported and understood at every step.

How to Develop Self-Discipline and Find Motivation

Setting goals is a commendable first step in fostering discipline and motivation. However, there are deeper, invaluable strategies to ensure you stay committed. Let's explore some compassionate pointers to fortify your self-discipline in this post-pandemic world.

1. Dive Deep into Your Motivations:

Understanding what fuels your passion is paramount. Ask yourself: What excites you? What drives your core? Recognizing these elements can act as a compass, guiding you toward activities and tasks you naturally gravitate towards.

"When was the last time you took the time to write down what you wanted? I had never done it until a couple of years ago; I first wrote about overcoming these anxious feelings."

2. Embrace What's Within Your Control:

Given the global challenges, it's understandable that some things weigh heavy on your mind. Yet, it's crucial to focus on the elements within your grasp. Accept that while adversities are a part of life, your reaction to them is within your control.

4 C's – Cause, Control, Cure, Contribute. *"If you find your thoughts leaning on something, then if you can't control or cure it, didn't cause or contribute to it, let it go."*

3. Lean on Motivating Quotes:

Whenever doubt or negativity creeps in, remind yourself of uplifting quotes. Mistakes are a part of growth. Remember, it's okay to falter; how you pick yourself up matters.

"There are daily readers of motivational quotes; treat yourself. You deserve it!"

4. Adopt a One-Word Mantra:

Phrases like "You're enough," "Embrace growth today," or "I Love You" while looking in the mirror (*trust me, that's a tough one!*) can make a world of difference. These one-word motivators can be your anchor on challenging days.

"Mine, every day, in every way, I'm getting better and better!"

5. Commit to Daily Routines:

Self-discipline is a journey, not a destination. It's about fostering habits over time. Celebrate small milestones and remember that self-care is equally crucial.

"Plan your healthy meals ahead of time."

6. Set Achievable Milestones:

Break down your goals. Starting with smaller, more manageable tasks can boost your confidence and pave the way for more significant achievements.

"Goals are like steps; once you recognize you have completed the first step, the second is and can be more manageable."

7. Draw Inspiration from Your Surroundings:

Motivation is everywhere. Take a moment to reflect on your successes, no matter how minute. Likewise, draw encouragement from the triumphs of those around you.

"Inspiration can indeed be found in another's accomplishments. Be present and observe all the little magnificent happenings in your environment."

8. Don't Let Fear Hinder Your Success:

Fear of success, sometimes called impostor syndrome, can be as debilitating as fear of failure. Remember, you're continually evolving. Embrace the change.

"Affirm that you are worthy; if you aspire to become an author, for example, affirm "I am an author." You'll be amazed at the results."

Understanding Motivation:

Motivation isn't just an abstract concept; it's the fuel that drives action. And contrary to popular belief, motivation often follows action, not vice versa.

"So, the key? Take Action and Just start! Live the life you've imagined!"

The Ritual of Motivation:

Cultivate daily rituals that prompt action. Begin with simple acts that naturally transition you into your main task. Over time, these small beginnings create momentum, propelling you forward.

"First thing in the morning, think of one thing you are grateful for."

Maintaining Long-Term Motivation:

To stay motivated, find challenges that are just right—not too difficult, yet not too simple. This "Goldilocks Rule" ensures you're always engaged and motivated.

"Set one daily goal, small but adequate and revisit it at the end of the day—check in with yourself."

When motivation starts to wane—and it might—it's crucial to revisit your goals and adjust as needed. Life is a journey of continuous recalibration. Even if you're only taking small steps, you're moving forward. Celebrate that bravery and that effort and know that every step counts. You've got this.

RELATABLE STORIES

- "Block scheduling has worked tons for me. Planning my week on Sunday has helped a ton as well. Having mental clarity about what I want to accomplish and why I want to do it has helped me become more consistent. I like to shoot for the stars and then re-evaluate and

readjust based on the week's results," (TheRealLex43, 2021).
- "Whatever you need to do, put it in a schedule. So, figure out when it's time to do this thing, and put it in your calendar, setting up reminders that tell you when it's time. For your exercise plan, establish when you'll be exercising, where you'll do it, what materials you'll need, and how long this will go on," (brenthuras, 2021).
- "Sometimes, what really pushes me and puts me in a state of urgency is asking myself or telling myself, 'Do I want to stay in the same spot until I'm 40?', 'Am I going to keep doing the same things and having the same habits in 20 years?'" (mabdel511, 2021).

You've acquired insights into combating procrastination and mastered techniques to sustain motivation. Remember, motivation is deeply personal. What fuels one person's passion might not resonate with another. It's vital to honor your unique motivational triggers, permanently anchoring them in your beliefs, interests, and aspirations. As you further hone the wisdom and skills you've gathered, let's take a moment to recognize your incredible capacity for growth and transformation. The next chapter will delve deeper into embracing sustainable progress, helping you flourish in the evolving post-pandemic landscape.

7

EMBRACING SUSTAINABLE GROWTH AND THRIVING

 Don't go through life, grow through life.

— ERIC BUTTERWORTH

As you take that pivotal step away from the profound impact of the pandemic and our global calamity, you'll find the essence of embracing change and thriving in this new normal to be more crucial than ever. The shifts the pandemic thrust upon you are not just challenges but invitations to adapt and re-evaluate what truly matters in your life. As you stand on the precipice of what's next, realize that you possess the remarkable opportunity to craft a resilient and sustainable future for yourself and your loved ones.

When you open your heart to a growth mindset, the barriers before you transform into stepping stones of knowledge and self-improvement. Imagine choosing growth over stagnation every single day, channeling the anxiety and apprehension into drive and creativity. This way of thinking doesn't just help you cope with the uncertainties of a post-pandemic world but empowers you to thrive amidst them as they unfold and evolve.

This is your chance, your canvas. Reimagine your life, your community, and the broader world with a lens focused on sustainability and collective wellness. You've weathered storms before; we all have. So why not tap into that innate power within you to create a brighter, more hopeful future? Together, let's sculpt a world that resonates with empathy and collective strength through the common denominator of love.

Sustained growth and prosperity? It's rooted in the habits you cultivate, the consistency you maintain, and the never-ending thirst for learning. You're building momentum toward your dreams with each consistent action and beneficial habit. Let the growth mindset be your North Star, redirecting every challenge into an opportunity and fortifying your resilience. This is your strategy for success that stands the test of time. Remember the **'E' in the B-BRAVE framework?** It's your beacon of hope and optimism. Embrace it.

CONSISTENCY AND HABITS

Consistency is the heartbeat of habit formation. Imagine setting small, achievable targets and steadily working towards them. Just as continuous unfavorable actions can spiral into detrimental habits—like reaching for that midnight snack or snoozing the alarm one too many times—couldn't the same persistence carve out positive habits too?

The Power of Consistency

You've set dreams and goals for yourself, but they can only materialize through persistent effort. Dreaming of a restful night's sleep isn't enough. It's the repeated act of settling into bed early and rising with the dawn that makes it second nature. Such consistency shapes your habits, refining them until they blend seamlessly into your daily rhythm. Remember, success isn't just about envisioning, it's taking intentional strides toward it.

"One can show an intention to another through action and non-action."

Habit Formation through Consistency

Embrace the understanding that transformation doesn't happen overnight. It demands resilience, granting you the tenacity to push forward, even when the road gets tough. Reflect on the 'why' behind your desire for change. Perhaps your erratic sleep pattern has been the unseen culprit shadowing your personal and professional life. Recognizing this, your inner drive kicks in, propelling you towards healthier routines.

Guiding Steps to Habitual Consistency

1. **Prioritize Yourself:** Change for you, not for anyone else. Let your growth and goals stem from a deep-seated desire for self-betterment. Block out external voices and tune into your inner motivations.
2. **Stay Connected to Your "Why":** Surround yourself with reminders of the reasons behind your change. Sticky notes on mirrors, alerts on your phone, or daily affirmations can serve as gentle nudges. Usually, after a few weeks, the efforts start to become second nature.
3. **Seek Companionship:** Find a kindred spirit or join a support group. Sharing your journey with someone on a similar path can be incredibly motivating. They're not just companions; they're mirrors reflecting mutual progress and encouragement.
4. **Celebrate Progress, Not Perfection:** Expect a winding path, not a straight one. If you slip up one day, give yourself grace and start afresh the next. Each step, no matter how small, brings you closer to your goal.

Embrace the journey, cherishing each moment of growth and self-discovery. Remember, it's not about how quickly you achieve your goals but the resilience and passion with which you pursue them.

"Life is a journey, not a destination, so enjoy the journey!"

GROWTH AND LEARNING

Ever since you were a child, you've had a passion for reading, or you may have not. You'd let your mind wander, dreaming of becoming one of those legendary authors whose names resonate across the globe or just being the best in your trade or skill. But, just like others, you might have believed in the limiting narrative that some destinies are just set in stone. You might've heard whispers like, "I'm just not cut out to be an athlete," or "I don't have the brains to be a mathematician." If such unwritten rules applied, then perhaps pursuing dreams of authorship seemed like chasing the wind. The world, as you perceived it, was divided: there were iconic authors like Stephen King and Agatha Christie, and then there was the "rest" of us.

Maybe, for a while, you accepted being in the ranks of the "ordinary." But then something shifted. The discovery of a growth mindset illuminated a new path. The realization that change is not just possible but within one's grasp became evident. Clinging to beliefs that limit growth can be detrimental. But here's the truth you've come to embrace: Your destiny is yours to shape, and no mindset should ever hinder your aspirations. Your potential is boundless, and who you wish to become is entirely up to you. Dive into that belief and watch how transformation unfolds.

Why a Growth Mindset Is Essential

When you were a child, you learned essential skills that prepared you for adulthood, like walking, speaking, and understanding numbers and words. But why, upon reaching adulthood, might you feel as if the door to learning new skills has suddenly closed? Let me assure you, it hasn't. You have the innate ability to continually learn and adapt to new situations.

With a growth mindset, you won't be trapped by doubts that question your intelligence or abilities. Instead, you'll be driven by the desire for progress, focusing on goals that enrich and elevate you. Maybe writing wasn't your strength a decade ago but you believe in your potential for growth. With dedication and practice, just imagine where you could be. Embrace this journey with compassion for yourself and see how far you can truly go.

"If your growth doesn't scare you, dig deeper, chase that far-reaching dream, and be a unique you!"

How to Make Sure You Keep Growing and Learning

The saying "experience is the best teacher" rings true, doesn't it? You might find, as many do, that the richest lessons come from lived experiences and an insatiable hunger for growth. Whenever you harbor a desire to uncover new horizons, rest assured you're on a path of continuous learning. By embracing this journey, you're not just learning but evolving into the best version of yourself.

Here's a gentle nudge with some insights that might guide you on this quest for personal growth:

Cultivating the Right Mindset:

Relying solely on innate talents can sometimes be limiting. Remember, nurturing a growth mindset can be transformative.

As you journey, be mindful of this perspective, and celebrate the little strides you make. It's through recognizing your progress that you'll find the zest to move forward.

"Be present, reward yourself; after all, you deserve it; trust me, it's not selfish!"

Embrace Learning Goals:

Ever paused to reflect on patterns or habits that might be holding you back? Setting specific learning intentions can be enlightening. It gives you clarity, helping you spot any mindset traps or behaviors that might be creating ripples in your personal or professional world. By identifying these, you can chart a course for growth.

"Understand your hungry ghosts when they arrive; yes, to sabotage your goal, don't feed them."

Heed the Signals of Today:

Sometimes, discomfort can be a guide. Maybe there was a time when a chat with friends turned unexpectedly tense. Reflect on that. Were you perhaps dominating the conversation? It's these moments of introspection that unveil opportunities for growth. For instance, realizing the importance of balanced exchanges ensures that everyone feels seen and heard in a conversation.

"Be present with your feelings, allow them, yet don't allow them to control the outcome of a conversation; after all, it's a pivotal point in growing; the first step is to congratulate yourself; you recognized it".

Cherish Future Aspirations:

Dreams and fantasies can be profound motivators. Picture where you hope to be a few years from now. Whether it's envisioning a flourishing business, mastering a craft, reaching a career pinnacle, or overcoming fear and anxiety, let these dreams steer you. For example, if you dream of becoming a renowned author, even if you start with modest writing skills, let that vision inspire you. With every word you pen, you're a step closer to that dream.

"Embark on this journey of self-discovery with kindness to yourself, and watch as every experience shapes you, molds you, and elevates you."

Phantoms of the Past

Childhood is often where you first shape your understanding of the world. Some lessons uplift you, while others might confine you. The roles, identities, values, and beliefs instilled in you by your family play a profound role in shaping your actions as you step into adulthood. This deeply rooted identity, the inner child, so closely held, can influence your behaviors, sometimes making it challenging to evolve, even when you strive for change.

Growing up, were you taught to be fiercely independent, to face challenges head-on without seeking help? Did it ever feel like you were expected to bear your burdens alone, without the luxury of reaching out or leaning on someone else? Picture this: as an adult, a close friend confides in you about their relationship troubles. Instead of offering a listening ear, you might've said, "Don't dwell on it. It's not a big deal." Such a response, while unintended, can inadvertently minimize their feelings.

Reflecting on these moments, you might recognize the unintentional harm in being dismissive when someone reaches out. But every realization is an opportunity for growth. Your evolving goal? To become adept at both offering and receiving support, to genuinely acknowledge the struggles of others, and to respond with empathy and encouragement.

"For many years, I carried the weight of unresolved issues, holding onto them like phantoms. Despite the passage of time, I refused to give up on understanding the early wounds inflicted upon me. I recognized that my mother, operating at her own level of growth and trying to protect me, did her best. Her message was clear: You show more contempt by saying nothing. I held this message during my younger years, opting to suppress my feelings of pain and anger. I thought that by doing so, I would be exhibiting contempt rather than addressing my emotions. These patterns impacted my life, affecting my relationships and businesses. I became a 'yes man,' missing out on many opportunities because I failed to express my opinions."

Conduct Experiments

Conducting experiments is about broadening your horizons and stepping out of your comfort zone. You might wonder why you'd ever venture beyond what's familiar. The answer is simple: embracing new experiences paves the way for unexpected discoveries. Even if a path seems unrelated to your ultimate goal, walking it can offer invaluable lessons. Consider wanting to become a successful author. Beyond mastering the craft of writing, there's a world of knowledge awaiting you, from understanding the intricacies of publishing to expanding your network. Remember, every tiny step is a significant stride toward your dreams.

Feedback can be a powerful catalyst for growth. While it's natural to be hesitant, fearing criticism or judgment, know that embracing feedback demonstrates your commitment to improvement. Others will see this as a sign of your genuine interest in learning and evolving. After all, growth often emerges from moments of discomfort; learn to be uncomfortable.

And as you forge ahead, keep a few strategies in mind:

1. **Harness the Power of the Internet.** The digital world is bursting with opportunities to learn about new hobbies, recreational activities, and anything your heart desires for the most part. Engage yourself in that something you've always wanted to do.
2. **Dive into Volunteering.** While these roles might not always come with a paycheck, they offer rich learning experiences. Volunteering can help you expand your skills and connect with like-minded individuals.
3. **Engage in Workshops and Seminars.** With the rise of virtual events, it's easier than ever to join discussions, workshops, and seminars. Here, you'll find fresh insights and the chance to interact with others having similar challenges.

Remember, every experience, every piece of feedback, and every new learning opportunity is a step closer to your aspirations. Embrace them with an open mind and heart.

 "You're not everything you could be, and you know it."

— DR. JORDAN B. PETERSON

RELATABLE STORIES

- "My only tip is to focus on what you want. I remained jobless for four years. I was asking everyone to help me hunt for a job but got no help. After four years, I planned to focus on my career. Bought a course from Udemy and started learning Digital Marketing. Completed the course in a month and applied for a job. Got the job in the first month as an intern. After four years, now I'm standing in a position that I never thought of," (ResearchWithAnna, 2021).
- Imagine various people from your life speaking at your funeral–this might include your parents, spouse, coworkers, or friends. What do you want them to say about you? When I performed this exercise, I realized that I wanted people to remember me as loving and supportive, inspirational, and hard-working to provide hope and alleviate suffering both in my local and global

community, etc. I wrote these things down, and it eventually evolved into my Personal Mission Statement—a series of bullet points that summarize the values I want to embody in my daily life," (TheAnonymousHippo, 2021).

- "Problems are good. Problems indicate growth. You become a new person whenever you overcome a problem. The real problem is that you're not excited about your problems! The next time you're faced with a problem, convince your brain that this is a good thing!" (SirNerdRomeo, 2021).

Continuous growth through life's experiences is vital for navigating our ever-evolving world. You need to remain open to acquiring new skills, leveraging technology in beneficial ways, embracing feedback from those around you, and fostering a growth mindset. By embracing these strategies, you're not just staying afloat; you're positioning yourself at the forefront of progress and success.

With the completion of the **B-BRAVE framework,** you've equipped yourself with invaluable tools to refine your mindset and harness techniques to transform life's challenges into fuel for growth and self-betterment. It's not just an achievement; it's a profound journey of self-evolution. Celebrate this transformative journey, recognizing the incredible strides you've made.

Who Are You! If you still can't answer the question, work on it, B-BRAVE!

8

CELEBRATING YOUR JOURNEY OF PERSONAL TRANSFORMATION

> *Life is a moving, breathing thing. We have to be willing to constantly evolve. Perfection is constant transformation.*
>
> — NIA PEEPLES

Your personal transformation is a journey worth celebrating. No matter how seemingly insignificant, each stride you take is a testament to your ability to evolve and grow. This journey is an invitation to get closer to your true self to embrace a life that resonates deeply with who you are. Embrace this transformative power that resides within you.

To truly harness this transformation, it's vital for you to cultivate gratitude. This practice isn't just a feel-good exercise; it's a tool to bolster your confidence and resilience. By cherishing your milestones and focusing on the positive shifts in your life, you're equipping yourself with an optimistic lens, especially crucial in a world reshaped by the repercussions of the pandemic and an ever-evolving world.

But understanding change and feeling grateful is just the beginning. Setting fresh intentions and resolutions, coupled with the determination to see them through, often needs a refined approach. In this chapter, I'll walk beside you, helping you recognize your achievements, craft new ambitions, and inspire unwavering growth. It's simply the sensible path on this transformative journey. Dive in with an open mind and heart, and let's navigate this together.

EMBRACING GRATITUDE AND JOY

What if I told you that the secret to happiness lies in gratitude? Achieving true contentment might be simpler than you've imagined. By cultivating a mindset centered on gratitude, you have the power to discover joy in life's every moment.

Gone are the times when pristine report cards defined your worth or when you relied on constant validation from others to feel a sense of accomplishment. Genuine happiness and gratitude are right there, waiting for you to recognize them.

In this section, we'll delve deep into the transformative power of gratitude. I'll guide you through techniques and practices that will help you fully embrace the happiness you deserve, wrapping you in warmth and understanding every step of the way.

What Is Gratitude, and Why Is It Important?

During the pandemic, wasn't it challenging for you to find that glimmer of hope amidst the chaos? The world seemed to spiral out of control with the relentless stream of news about increasing cases and heart-wrenching losses. It might have felt like the beauty in life had dimmed, that the joy and elation you once knew seemed distant and elusive. As these challenging years unfolded, perhaps you, too, sensed the deep mental and emotional toll they took.

In the face of overwhelming adversity, it's only human to fixate on the negatives. Yet, it's crucial to remember that there's a ray of light for every shadow, and for every moment of despair, there exists the potential for happiness, gratitude, and joy.

When was the last time you relished a genuine moment of happiness, those cherished memories that warm your heart and bring a smile to your face? Maybe it was when you achieved a personal milestone or celebrated a loved one's special day. Remember, happiness isn't just a thing of the past. It's also a choice you can make right now, in this very moment, by acknowledging and cherishing the blessings that surround you, no matter how small.

Consider this: You still have a safe haven to return to, tantalizing meals that nourish you, and the health and vigor to embrace each new day. When you lean into gratitude, it can light up your world, even when times seem their darkest. That's the transformative power of gratitude: anchoring us in contentment and appreciation, especially when the horizon seems uncertain.

The Psychology of Gratitude and Happiness

Practicing gratitude has significant psychological advantages, as it allows individuals and a larger group of people to recognize the importance of maintaining a positive mindset. Extensive research focuses on the connection between positive behaviors and emotional well-being, revealing fascinating insights. Together, we can delve into these compassionate scientific findings and better understand how embracing gratitude can lead to genuine happiness.

Research in This Topic

Imagine discovering a simple, profound way to increase your happiness and strengthen your mental resilience. Practicing gratitude draws your focus to the positive moments, making you cherish the beauty in life's little moments. This simple act isn't just about feeling good in the moment; it's a long-term investment in your mental well-being.

Back in 2001, Danner and his team carried out a fascinating study centered on gratitude and how it might affect longevity. They chose nuns from across the U.S., a group selected for their shared lifestyles, diets, and religious routines. These nuns penned essays, sharing their life stories, dreams, and aspirations. When the researchers revisited these essays after some years, they found an inspiring correlation: nearly 90% of the nuns who wove gratitude into their tales lived past the age of 85.

In another compelling study by Emmons and McCullough in 2003, participants journaled weekly, focusing on varied topics—from daily blessings to daily irritations. Ten weeks later, the findings were uplifting: those who had poured out gratitude and hope in their writings not only felt emotionally more balanced but also had fewer medical visits.

So, as you journey through life seeking happiness, remember this: embedding gratitude in your daily routine might not just be a path to joy but a cornerstone to building a richer, fuller life. Dive deep into gratitude, and watch as it transforms not only your day but perhaps even your life's trajectory.

From my own journey, I've deeply felt the power of gratitude. When my mother was diagnosed with breast cancer, her unwavering attitude of gratitude and determination that cancer wouldn't defeat her gifted us, her children, with an additional 15 precious years with her.

How Does Gratitude Bring Happiness?

So, science has shown us that gratitude can lead to a longer life, but how does it directly influence your sense of happiness?

When you adopt positive mindsets such as optimism, joy, and vigor, your lifespan can truly extend. By integrating gratitude into your daily routine, you deepen your connection to uplifting thoughts and feelings, enabling you to navigate life's ups and downs with grace and resilience. But gratitude isn't solely about relishing in happy moments; it's a bridge to forming profound, meaningful bonds with others and, importantly, with yourself.

By nurturing relationships rooted in authentic conversations, mutual trust, and enhanced self-esteem, you don't just elevate your own happiness. You also strengthen the ties that bind you to others. Let gratitude be your guiding light, casting a warm glow on pathways of connection, support, and genuine joy in your life.

Does Gratitude Multiply Happiness?

Absolutely! When you cultivate gratitude, you're nurturing positive emotions within yourself. These emotions become a safeguard, protecting you from negative thoughts that might otherwise lead you down challenging paths. Even in moments where daunting thoughts arise, you possess the strength to set them aside and let your true capabilities shine.

Through gratitude, you learn to navigate life's storms with grace, taking each situation in stride without draining your valuable mental and emotional energy. It's in this practice of acceptance that you truly understand resilience, giving yourself the compassion you deserve as you journey through life's highs and lows.

While working at a hardware store years ago, the atmosphere was rather sad. Was it the vibe of the staff in the store or my feelings contributing to my growing aversion to showing up? Something had to change. Taking deliberate steps, though gradual, I began to cultivate gratitude towards my customers, who, in essence, provided my paycheck and appreciated my uplifting personality. This shift didn't go unnoticed. Colleagues began wondering about the newfound positivity I exuded, especially since I no longer let their disgruntled sentiments affect me. It raised the question: did my small steps in practicing gratitude transform my happiness and influence those around me? Yes, the proof is in the pudding.

Ways to Practice Gratitude

It's obvious that practicing gratitude will give us plenty of benefits. Now, how do we practice it? There are several exercises you can try. Below, I want to share common methods to be more grateful.

Gratitude Exercises

- Meditation stands out as a profound method to embrace gratitude. As you might recall from our earlier discussions, meditation can heighten your awareness of the present moment and help balance your emotions. Remember chapter four? Revisit it to refresh your understanding of cultivating mindfulness and cherishing the countless blessings in your life.
- Have you ever tried gratitude mapping? It's a heartfelt way to visualize all that you're thankful for. Imagine crafting a mind map or a mood board brimming with positive emotions and elements of your life that fill your heart with gratitude. Once created, position it somewhere you frequently see—perhaps your bedroom or living area. Let it be a daily nudge, a gentle reminder of the abundance in your life.
- Consider jotting down your moments of gratitude on small slips of paper. As you fold them, place each one in

a jar. Over time, these jars become reservoirs of your gratitude, brimming with memories and reminders.

Every note is a testament that no matter the day, there's always a silver lining, always something to cherish.

Gratitude Prompts

When navigating the complexities of life, it's vital for you to find moments of gratitude that anchor your spirit. Reflect on the beauty found in the simplest pleasures: that comforting cup of morning tea or a cherished song that brightens your day. Cherish the memories that remind you of happiness—those gatherings with loved ones, birthday celebrations, or just a random joyful day. Think of the friends, family, and colleagues who've stood by you, offering support through life's highs and lows. Let nature be your sanctuary; relish the tranquility of a rainy day or the warmth of the sun on your face. Remember to express your gratitude, both in feeling and in action. Every "thank you" shared, every act of kindness you extend, amplifies the value you see in the world around you. Celebrate your achievements, no matter how big or small, and jot them down as a testament to your journey. Amidst the hustle, find a serene moment just for yourself, breathe in deeply, and let gratitude fill your heart for the present moment.

Gratitude Journals

The most profound way to immerse yourself in gratitude is by penning down the things you're grateful for in a journal. Think of it as a personal diary where you reflect on the day's experiences and highlight the moments of gratitude.

You might find it comforting to jot down your feelings of gratitude two to three times a week. Using bullet lists can be an incredibly grounding technique, allowing you to quickly note down those treasures of thankfulness. Remember, your journal entries don't need to be lengthy narratives; even a few heartfelt words can serve as gentle reminders of life's blessings.

To ease you into this journey of gratitude journaling, here are some prompts and a template to inspire and guide your writing. Embrace this opportunity; it's a gentle nudge toward recognizing and celebrating the good in your world.

Gratitude Journal Template

- What unfolded in your day today? Reflect and jot down some of the activities that marked your hours.
- Where did you find moments of joy? Let your heart trace back to those instants that kindled happiness or evoked a smile. Even a short list of three to five such moments can be deeply revealing. Sometimes, it's the simplest things that shine the brightest.
- Pause for a moment and ponder: What would leave an empty space in your heart if it were to vanish? Put pen to paper and capture those treasured things or cherished individuals that you hold close. Remember, it's these very elements that often give our days meaning and warmth.

"You can do an awful lot by writing down what happened to you and thinking it through."

— DR. JORDAN B. PETERSON

SETTING NEW GOALS AND CONTINUED GROWTH

Have you ever set New Year's resolutions, only to find them untouched and forgotten as the months roll by? Those lingering promises on your list, patiently waiting for the moment when you muster the willpower to begin. Each year, you might think, "This year will be different," and fervently jot down your aspirations. Yet, only a few weeks later, they're tucked away and forgotten.

Why does reaching our goals seem so elusive? When these ambitions mean so much, why do we sometimes overlook the significance of steady progress and meticulous planning? As you delve deeper, you might realize that goal setting goes beyond simply penning down optimistic visions of a "new you." For true transformation, it's essential to understand where you currently stand and chart your progress.

In this section, let's compassionately explore the profound impact of goal setting and discover the most effective ways to chase and achieve those dreams.

On a bitterly cold day in February, I found myself standing on the front porch, nursing a terrible cold, yet inexplicably lighting a cigarette. Holding it, I questioned myself deeply, "Why am I doing this?" Some might think I was out of my mind. In that moment of clarity, I extinguished my cigarette, walked inside, and threw the entire pack into the trash, choosing to quit cold turkey. It was far from easy; the pull of nicotine is relentless.

However, whenever I felt a craving, I grounded myself in the present, understanding it was just a temporary urge from a long-held habit. It's truly a battle of mind over matter. Conquering that challenge filled me with newfound confidence. I genuinely believe that if I could overcome that, I—or anyone—can achieve anything they set their mind to.

The Importance and Value of Goal Setting

Over the years, have you found yourself disheartened by the goals you've set, only to leave them by the wayside later? What's the point of these aspirations if they no longer resonate with your heart? Sometimes, it might feel like jotting down these objectives adds another weight to your shoulders—an additional challenge to face. You long for personal growth, so why does goal setting occasionally seem counterproductive?

Yet, setting intentions can be a powerful motivator, ushering in fresh habits and new perspectives. The daunting nature of this task stems from not truly understanding how to gauge your progress or grasp the true essence of setting these markers. For you to harness the transformative power of goals, it's vital to recognize their inherent value and the profound impact they can have on your journey.

Why Set Goals in Life?

I understand that many of you struggle with staying committed to your goals. Simply jotting down aspirations on paper and hoping they'll materialize isn't the essence of effective goal setting. It's about pinpointing a clear objective and charting a course to achieve it. And I know reaching goals can be tough and sometimes disheartening. This is why it's essential to differentiate between a genuine, purposeful goal and a fleeting wish for self-improvement.

If you set a goal like "be more active," ask yourself: what true motivation does that offer you? While it's an aspiration, does it truly inspire commitment? Instead of moving aimlessly, why not target something tangible you desire? Consider opting for "participate in and complete a marathon." This not only gives you a clear aim but necessitates a specific training regimen.

By choosing such a goal, you take command of your life's direction. You dictate the actions and commitments of your upcoming weeks or months, aligning them with the marathon objective. Such a goal doesn't just motivate you momentarily; it paints a vivid picture of the person you aspire to become. This is the genuine power of goal setting: it bestows upon you a profound sense of purpose.

My "why" began with an overwhelming weariness from the anxious ebbs and flows that dominated my life. I committed to grappling with those feelings, and just before the pandemic, I felt I had finally achieved some semblance of equilibrium. But then, the onslaught of COVID-19 catapulted my anxieties to unparalleled heights. Each day, I donned my mask, a symbolic veneer, venturing into the world while concealing the turmoil within. Was this charade genuinely worth it? Trapping those emotions inside what I imagined as a "genie bottle" served neither me nor those around me. The bottled-

up emotions, rather than disappearing, simply waited for release.

WHAT ARE THE BENEFITS OF GOAL SETTING?

Setting goals isn't just about checking boxes or achieving milestones; it's about nurturing your journey toward self-fulfillment and clarity. When you set a goal, you're not just laying out a plan; you're giving yourself direction, a purpose. Each goal offers you mental clarity, pinpointing what you truly desire. It becomes a beacon, lighting up your path with motivation, enabling you to embrace growth.

Have you ever felt the pure satisfaction that comes from achieving something you once deemed challenging? *I have!* That's the magic of setting clear and challenging goals. They might stretch you, but in that stretch, you'll find growth, discovery, and an exhilarating sense of accomplishment. And with every goal you set, remember to commit to it, seek feedback, and understand that some goals, especially complex ones, require patience. Embrace the journey they offer.

But there's more. The very act of setting a goal can uplift your performance. When you aim high, the challenge propels you to strive harder, resulting in remarkable improvements. This heightened performance doesn't just boost productivity; it's a reflection of your evolving confidence, a testament to your understanding of your own capabilities. Imagine the wonders this newfound self-belief can do for your family and professional life.

Moreover, consider the lasting motivation that accompanies

effective goal setting. Researchers Locke and Latham suggest that when you use goals as your benchmarks and seek feedback, it not only fuels your current aspirations but kindles long-term motivation. It's like lighting a fire within that keeps you warm and illuminated throughout your journey.

And in the realm of mental well-being, goal setting takes on an even more profound role. Picture this: adults grappling with depression, finding solace and improvement through the simple act of setting personal goals. A study resonated with this very sentiment, highlighting how goal setting can elevate the desire for personal growth, magnify the longing to get better and intensify the courage to seek help. Just having one person support you with accountability check-ups helps keep the goal alive and very attainable.

So, as you navigate life's intricate maze, remember the transformative power of goal setting. It's not just a task; it's a compass, a motivator, a healer, and, most importantly, a beacon of hope and growth for you.

Determining Your Goals

Begin by reflecting on your passions, core values, and interests to define your goals. Ask yourself what truly ignites your spirit and drives your enthusiasm. Perhaps, like many, you're drawn to a deeper understanding of yourself. Maybe anxiety or other emotions prompt you to seek knowledge and skills to help you understand their roots. Think about the legacy you want to leave and the impact you wish to have on your local or the more extensive global community. These reflections can be powerful catalysts in setting meaningful goals for your life.

In the following sections, I'm eager to share compassionate strategies to help guide you in pinpointing your goals and charting a course to your dreams. Dive in, and let's embark on this transformative journey together.

How to Set Goals in Seven Steps

You've been there, haven't you? Setting numerous goals, only to find yourself walking away before seeing even a hint of progress, or perhaps not even embarking on the journey at all. It's okay. It might indicate that your approach to goal setting needs a little fine-tuning. Achieving a dream requires more than sheer determination; it combines strategy, heart, and dedication. Let's navigate together through a seven-step method to set goals in a way that resonates deeply with who you are.

Step One: Visualize the Outcome

Imagine your aspirations. Visualize the results. How would accomplishing this goal enrich your life? Before taking that leap, immerse yourself in the potential rewards. Ponder on the transformations you'd experience and the person you'd evolve into once you cross the finish line.

Step Two: Embrace SMART Goals

You might've heard of the SMART framework; it's renowned for a reason. Ensure each goal you set resonates with these criteria:

- **Specific:** Be concise. Define your goal with clarity about what success looks like and why it matters to you.
- **Measurable:** Give your goal a quantifiable aspect. This helps in gauging progress and determining necessary adjustments.
- **Attainable:** Aim high but within the realms of possibility. Stretch yourself but remember to be grounded.
- **Realistic:** Your goals should be relevant, resonating with where you are in life. Ask yourself: Is this the right time for this particular aspiration?
- **Timely:** Infuse your goal with a sense of time. A defined timeline not only keeps you on track but fuels motivation.

Step Three: Put Pen to Paper

To breathe life into your dreams, jot them down. Place them where your eyes often wander—your workspace, bedside table, or even your phone's wallpaper. Let them serve as daily reminders of the path you've chosen.

Step Four: Chart Your Path

Having a goal is just the start. Sketch out your action plan—these are the stepping stones leading to your dream. For instance, if you dream of running a marathon, think about the training involved. Maybe it's time to join a gym or embrace the open roads for some long runs.

Step Five: Draft a Timeline

Segment your journey by setting specific checkpoints and deadlines. Having these markers can invigorate your efforts, reminding you of the progress you're making and the milestones yet to come.

Step Six: Step Forward with Purpose

Now's the time to dive in. With each step, remember you're not just moving closer to your goal; you're growing, evolving, and becoming.

Step Seven: Reflect and Realign

Pause periodically to assess. Celebrate your progress, no matter how small. Are you on track? Rejoice in your growth and allow it to propel you forward, inching closer to that cherished dream.

Remember, setting and working toward a goal is a journey of self-discovery, resilience, and evolution. Each step, each hurdle, and each success are a testament to your spirit. Embrace the process with compassion, understanding that you deserve every achievement that comes your way.

Ask Yourself Why

One of the most compassionate steps you can take when setting a goal is to gently ask yourself, "Why?" Why does this particular goal resonate with your heart? What internal pull drives you toward its realization? Taking a moment to truly reflect on these questions can unveil the deep-rooted purpose that anchors your aspirations. Such introspection can illuminate the value and richness these goals might bring to your near future, providing you with the heartfelt commitment to see them through. Truly understanding the tender motivations behind your goals helps ensure they resonate with your true essence, beautifully mirroring who you are and the dreams you cherish.

State Goals with a Positive Tone

Declare your goals with an uplifting and affirmative tone to ensure that your motivations stem from genuine and positive intentions. For instance, if your aim is to shed five pounds in a month, rather than stating, "I want to appear slim," consider expressing, "I aspire to embrace a healthier, more vibrant lifestyle." This shift in perspective not only deepens your connection with your intentions but also bolsters your confidence and trust in your capabilities. Remember, it's about embracing your journey with self-compassion and understanding, drawing strength from the reasons that truly resonate with your heart.

Focus on the Process, Not the Outcome

Setting a goal can often be the most challenging mindset to embrace. It's understandable that when you set an aspiration, your thoughts might become consumed by the anticipated outcome. However, homing in solely on the final result can sometimes overshadow the importance of the journey itself. If you fixate solely on the desire to lose 20 pounds in a month, there's a risk of overlooking the daily steps needed to get there. Instead of wholeheartedly adopting a balanced diet and a vibrant, active routine, the weight-loss number might loom too large, potentially hindering the genuine progress you could be making. Remember, the consistent, compassionate choices you make each day will lead to lasting transformation.

Make a Contract with Yourself

A personal contract serves as a guiding light, ensuring you remain true to the promises and commitments you set for yourself. Here are some compassionate suggestions to help you craft a contract that truly resonates with your innermost desires and aspirations:

- Envision and articulate your dreams and objectives.
- Reflect upon and list your inherent strengths.
- Recognize potential challenges or roadblocks that might stand in your path.
- Delineate the proactive measures you intend to take to navigate these hurdles.
- On a heartfelt scale of 1–10, gauge your genuine confidence in realizing your aspirations.

Once penned, take a deep breath and, with utmost sincerity, declare aloud: "I wholeheartedly commit to the intentions and strategies within this contract. Whenever doubts cloud my path, I will turn to this contract as a reminder of my unwavering commitment to my goals."

Clear Out the Old to Make Room for the New

Just as you would rejuvenate a workspace or revamp a home, clearing away old clutter and welcoming new elements can infuse your life with renewed purpose. When you set your sights on your goals, gently release any limiting beliefs or self-doubt that might be tethering you. Open your heart to the boundless possibilities ahead, center yourself on growth, and have faith in your innate capacity to realize your aspirations. Remember, you are deserving of every success you seek.

Seek Support

Seeking support when you set a goal can be a heartfelt way to ensure you're on the right path. Imagine drawing from the wisdom and guidance of those who've walked the journey before you. Envelop yourself in a community that uplifts and supports you because every step you take towards your goal is made easier with encouragement from those around you. Remember, achieving success isn't a solitary journey; reaching out for help can amplify your chances of flourishing. Embrace the journey, knowing you're not alone, and let the collective strength guide you.

REWARD YOURSELF

Rewarding yourself can be a powerful source of motivation. Always take a moment to recognize, appreciate, and honor your achievements as you journey toward your aspirations. Ensure your rewards are thoughtful, easily accessible, and frequent. For instance, after a rigorous workout, why not indulge in a few hours of relaxation? Maybe a rejuvenating nap or getting lost in the pages of a captivating book. Such acts of self-kindness not only bring immediate joy but also inspire continued progress, reminding you that you're deserving of every moment of self-care and celebration.

RELATABLE STORIES

- "Gratitude is not only the greatest of virtues but the parent of all others. I recommend applying this intergenerationally, as well. When you remember what people have given to create the world you live in, your duty to it does not seem so unreasonable or burdensome," (_olafr_, 2020).
- "Gratitude is focusing on all the good things in life and being thankful for everything that brings us happiness. It is about developing a thankful appreciation for all of life's joy and abundance instead of focusing on life's negative sides," (sickient, 2020).
- "I used to think that I was unable and incompetent. I thought I was just lazy, unmotivated, undisciplined, unfocused, and unhappy. Well, turns out that I was just

using the wrong strategies and tools. I'm still decades away from becoming my best self and achieving all my goals, but I'm on the correct trajectory. Because of self-development, I am now happier than ever, have a physique that I'm proud of, consistently develop my skills, have an ever-growing social circle, and am able to work for myself. You are only one breakthrough away from transforming your entire life. Stay persistent; stay on this path of self-development," (maxwesener, 2022).

Honoring your personal transformative journey is essential for your growth and development. It's crucial to acknowledge and cherish the strides you've made, the obstacles you've surpassed, and the invaluable lessons you've gathered along the way. Dive deep into gratitude and celebrate the progress you've achieved. Remember, each step you've taken is a testament to your strength and resilience.

INTERACTIVE ELEMENTS

In this section, you'll find interactive exercises crafted to deepen your understanding of the materials presented in this book. Each element is meticulously designed not just for your engagement but to spark reflection, urging you to delve deeper into the concepts rather than just skimming through them.

We'll journey through these exercises, mirroring the order of the B-BRAVE framework. It's my sincere hope that these activities help anchor your learning, immersing you more fully in the essence of this book. Dive in, engage in self-reflection, hone your problem-solving skills, and elevate your decision-making. Embrace this chance to transform knowledge into wisdom.

B: Banishing Fear, Worry, and Anxiety

In this exercise, practice self-acceptance and compassion by recognizing and feeling each negative emotion within you, then learn to accept them with an open mind.

Questions to Reflect	Answers
Feel each sensation in your body—your heart rate, breathing, and body temperature. Notice your doubts, questions, worries, and anxieties, then write them down.	<ul><li>_____</li><li>_____</li><li>_____</li><li>_____</li></ul>
Label your feelings and emotions. Do you feel worried, scared, or anxious? Write them down and describe your feelings briefly.	<ul><li>_____</li><li>_____</li><li>_____</li><li>_____</li><li>_____</li></ul>
Allow the experience to fill up your senses. Practice saying reassuring things to yourself (e.g., "It's okay to cry").	<ul><li>_____</li><li>_____</li><li>_____</li><li>_____</li></ul>
Respond to your emotions by reflecting and answering your questions and doubts. It's okay to say "I don't know" for each question you don't know the answer to.	<ul><li>_____</li><li>_____</li><li>_____</li><li>_____</li></ul>
Expand your awareness by connecting yourself with your environment. Be mindful of the present moment and list the things you're grateful for today.	<ul><li>_____</li><li>_____</li><li>_____</li><li>_____</li></ul>

B: Breaking Negative Thought Patterns

In this worksheet, practice acknowledging your automatic negative thoughts, learn to write them down, and learn how you can replace them with positive thoughts. Set aside some quiet time each day or each week for you to reflect on your negative thoughts.

Automatic Negative Thoughts	Positive Replacement Thoughts

R: Revising Core Beliefs

In this worksheet, practice identifying your negative core beliefs and try to find evidence that contradicts them.

What are your negative core beliefs?	List pieces of evidence contrary to your negative core beliefs.
I'm an unlikable person.	• I have friends who love me. • My family supports me. • I have a sibling who looks up to me.
What advice did your parents give that challenges your feelings?	• _____ • _____ • _____
	• _____ • _____ • _____
	• _____ • _____ • _____
	• _____ • _____ • _____
	• _____ • _____ • _____

A: Adopting Mindfulness

Refer to this simple checklist to help you get started on your mindfulness journey.

	Schedule a time and place for you to start practicing mindfulness meditation.
	Visit mindfulness communities and spaces around you.
	Keep a journal, notebook, or diary to write your feelings for the day.
	Say these words to yourself every day: "I am present now; I judge nothing."
	Pay attention to your thoughts, words, actions, and motivations.
	Dedicate a few minutes to take a break throughout the day.
	Don't think about the past, don't worry about the future, don't look at the time, just be.
	Notice your emotions and judgments and let them go.

V: Vanquishing Procrastination

In this worksheet, practice overcoming procrastination by reflecting and journaling about feelings, emotions, or distractions that influenced your procrastination. Write down the tasks that you avoid or postpone, then state your reasons.

Tasks You Avoid	Questions to Reflect
(Example: not doing homework.)	<ul><li>What excuses did you use?</li><li>What did you do instead of working?</li><li>What was the outcome?</li><li>What are your fears and worries?</li><li>What possible "procrastination triggers" can you identify?</li><li>What would happen if you didn't finish this task?</li></ul>

E: Embracing Sustainable Growth and Thriving

In this worksheet, practice identifying your habits (both good and bad), then try to change your negative habits.

Positive Habits	Negative Habits
1. (Example: practice meditating.)	1. (Example: eating junk food.)
2.	2.
3.	3.
4.	5.
6.	6.
7.	7.
8.	8.
9.	9.
10.	10.

Then, use the following activity to help break your negative habits.

What negative habits do you want to change? (e.g., eating junk food.)	• _____ • _____ • _____
What triggers these negative habits? (E.g., feeling stressed and wanting to eat junk food.)	• _____ • _____ • _____
How do you feel after doing these negative habits? (E.g., feeling satisfied after enjoying greasy and fatty food.)	• _____ • _____ • _____
What possible ways for you to break these negative habits? (E.g., bring healthy snacks when I'm outside, opt for healthier meals when eating outside.)	• _____ • _____ • _____ • _____
What words or situations trigger you? Where did they come from? (Can you relate this to a point in time from your childhood? If so, how did it hurt or affect you? Feel it and release it.)	• _____ • _____ • _____ • _____

Celebrating Your Journey of Personal Transformation

This is an informative daily exercise to assist in understanding how you are feeling and a precursor for goal setting. Use feeling words other than just good or bad. The morning section is a check-in for yourself, and the evening is your check-in on your progress. Be open and honest with yourself.

Morning	Monday	Tuesday	Wednesday	Thursday	Friday
Feeling Word for:					
Physical					
Mental					
Emotional					
Spiritual					
Goals: A goal to work on for the day and a skill to help you replace it.					
Skill					
Evening					
Strength					
Progress on your goal					
Barrier: what feelings did you experience					
Positive experience from your day					
Feeling					

As you complete the daily exercise above, you'll start fine-tuning your feelings and practicing your daily goal intentions; as I progressed, this exercise was very beneficial to my goal setting, leading me to the next worksheet.

In this worksheet, practice creating SMART goals and use them to reach your success.

   1. Write down your goals.

My goal is to…

   2. Make your goals **specific** and detailed. How will you reach this goal?

I will reach my goal by doing…

3. Make sure your goals are **measurable**. Write down your measurements and how you're going to track the progress.

I know I've achieved my goal when…

| |
| |
| |

4. Make your goals **attainable.** What resources do you need to achieve your goals?

I need to learn more about…

| |
| |
| |

5. Make your goals **relevant.** Why or how will your goals align with your life and your values?

This goal is important because…

6. Set the **time** to reach your goals.

I will reach my goal by… (write down the specific dates.)

CONCLUSION

Mastering your mindset isn't a final stop; it's a continuous journey, demanding dedication and leading to personal evolution, renewed positivity, and deepened self-compassion. As we reach the close of this book, reflect on the transformative power of a growth mindset, which is especially vital in a world forever changed by a profound pandemic.

You stand at a crucial juncture in history, navigating the realities of a post-pandemic era laden with challenges. Yet, beneath these layers of uncertainty, there exists a silver lining: the opportunity for self-betterment.

Throughout these pages, you've delved into the profound influence of mindset during unpredictable times. You've uncovered the necessity of nurturing mental resilience and embracing a growth mindset to flourish amidst adversity. The pandemic might have tested your mettle, but it also unveiled your potential to rise from setbacks. By confronting life's hurdles, you've learned to empower yourself, pushing past the shadows of fear, anxiety, and apprehension.

You've seen the beauty of positive reframing, the art of looking beyond obstacles to spot hidden opportunities. Together, we've dismantled self-limiting beliefs, tackled negative thought patterns, and replaced unconstructive core beliefs. You've gleaned insights on honing self-discipline, sustaining motivation, practicing mindfulness, and defeating procrastination. Think of these as foundational stones, essential in constructing a resilient mind.

To fortify these foundations, cherish every milestone, no matter how small, and immerse yourself in gratitude for the present. Such beliefs can sculpt your reality, ushering in positivity and influencing not just your actions but also those of the people around you.

Always remember: refining your mindset is an ongoing journey. Relish every moment of self-awareness, remain open to novel experiences, and never hesitate to seek assistance when the path seems daunting. As this chapter concludes, welcome the invigorating sense of purpose and joy it brings. Absorb the lessons to equip yourself for the awaiting horizons.

Embrace the wisdom from these pages and weave them into your daily life, ensuring success in our evolving world. Counter negative perceptions, welcome uncertainties, and practice mindfulness. Share your personal journey, enlightening your circle and the community. Perhaps consider initiating discussions that reinforce these principles, providing support to others on their own quests.

It's my sincere hope that the insights within these pages propel you toward continuous growth. Remember, nurturing a positive mindset isn't just beneficial—it's pivotal in sculpting a promising tomorrow. As you adapt to our new normal, do so with a renewed mindset.

Lastly, your feedback is invaluable. Sharing your reflections, critiques, or thoughts could inspire and guide another soul. Your perspective is not just welcomed—it's essential. Your story might be the beacon someone needs to chase away their darkness.

> "The secret to your existence is right in front of you. And it manifests itself as all those things you know you should do, but you're avoiding."
>
> — DR. JORDAN B. PETERSON

If you got inspired while reading and would like to continue receiving support and understanding, please join a group of like-minded individuals on Facebook
HEALTHY BODY - HEALTHY MIND
at CommonSenseFactor.us

C - Compassionate
O - Optimistic
M - Mindful
M - Motivated
O - Observant
N - Nurturing

S - Sincere
E - Empathetic
N - Nonjudgmental
S - Self-aware
E - Ethical

F - Forward-thinking
A - Adaptable
C - Cognizant
T - Tolerant
O - Objective
R - Resilient

REFERENCES

7 tactics for overcoming anxiety, by putting things into perspective. (2017, December 20). Psychology Compass. https://psychologycompass.com/blog/overcoming-anxiety/

10 Reasons why Consistency is important. (2021, August 9). Cabiojinia. https://cabiojinia.com/10-reasons-why-consistency-is-important/

American Psychological Association. (2021, October 19). *Demand for mental health treatment continues to increase, say psychologists.* Apa.org. https://www.apa.org/news/press/releases/2021/10/mental-health-treatment-demand

Ancona, D., & Perkins, D. N. T. (2022, January 1). *Family Ghosts in the Executive Suite.* Harvard Business Review. https://hbr.org/2022/01/family-ghosts-in-the-executive-suite

Andersen, C. H. (2023, January 9). *7 Simple Ways to Practice Gratitude in Your Everyday Life.* Reader's Digest. https://www.rd.com/article/how-to-practice-gratitude/

Anthony, K., & Wilson, D. R. (2017, December 1). *What Is EFT Tapping? 5-Step Technique for Anxiety Relief.* Healthline. https://www.healthline.com/health/eft-tapping#technique

Ash, T., & Silvestro, S. (2021, August 1). *12 Benefits Of Mindfulness For Mental and Physical Health.* Health Guide. https://ro.co/health-guide/12-benefits-of-mindfulness/

Ashford, S. J. (2022, September 28). *How to Make Sure You Keep Growing and Learning.* Greater Good. https://greatergood.berkeley.edu/article/item/how_to_make_sure_you_keep_growing_and_learning

Bailey, C. (2017, October 4). *5 Research-Based Strategies for Overcoming Procrastination.* Harvard Business Review. https://hbr.org/2017/10/5-research-based-strategies-for-overcoming-procrastination

Betterhelp Editorial Team. (2023, February 10). *Easy Ways To Incorporate Mindful Practices Into Daily Life | BetterHelp.* Www.betterhelp.com. https://www.betterhelp.com/advice/mindfulness/easy-ways-to-incorporate-mindful-practices-into-daily-life/

Bettino, K. (2021, June 2). *What's CBT and Is It Right for Me?* Psych Central.

https://psychcentral.com/lib/in-depth-cognitive-behavioral-therapy#how-it-works

Black, D. S., & Slavich, G. M. (2016). Mindfulness meditation and the immune system: a systematic review of randomized controlled trials. *Annals of the New York Academy of Sciences, 1373*(1), 13–24. https://doi.org/10.1111/nyas.12998

Bonati, M., Campi, R., & Segre, G. (2022). Psychological impact of the quarantine during the COVID-19 pandemic on the general European adult population: a systematic review of the evidence. *Epidemiology and Psychiatric Sciences, 31*. https://doi.org/10.1017/s2045796022000051

Booker, Z. (2023, February 9). *7 Ways to Keep Learning and Growing: Unleash Your Potential.* I4biz. https://www.i4biz.com/ways-to-keep-learning-and-growing/

Calbi, M., Langiulli, N., Ferroni, F., Montalti, M., Kolesnikov, A., Gallese, V., & Umiltà, M. A. (2021). The consequences of COVID-19 on social interactions: an online study on face covering. *Scientific Reports, 11*(1). https://doi.org/10.1038/s41598-021-81780-w

Casabianca, S. S., & Gepp, K. (2021, July 29). *Can You Stop Negative Thoughts by Changing Cognitive Distortions?* Psych Central. https://psychcentral.com/lib/fixing-cognitive-distortions#takeaway

Celestine, N. (2015, November 24). *How Psychology Combats False & Self-Limiting Beliefs.* PositivePsychology.com. https://positivepsychology.com/false-beliefs/

Cherry, K. (2021, April 29). *Why Cultivating a Growth Mindset Can Boost Your Success.* Verywell Mind. https://www.verywellmind.com/what-is-a-mindset-2795025

Cherry, K. (2022a, September 2). *What are the benefits of mindfulness?* Verywell Mind. https://www.verywellmind.com/the-benefits-of-mindfulness-5205137

Cherry, K. (2022b, November 14). *What Is Procrastination?* Verywell Mind. https://www.verywellmind.com/the-psychology-of-procrastination-2795944#toc-causes

Chopra, D. (2017, September 15). *Present-Moment Awareness: A Better Way to Stay in Control.* Chopra. https://chopra.com/articles/present-moment-awareness-a-better-way-to-stay-in-control

ChronWell. (2022, July 19). *Long-Term Effects of the Pandemic on Mental Health.* ChronWell. https://www.chronwell.com/long-term-effects-of-the-pandemic-on-mental-health/

Clear, J. (2015). *Motivation: The Scientific Guide on How to Get and Stay Motivated.* James Clear. https://jamesclear.com/motivation

Cornain, E. (2020, May 4). *The New Normal: How life has changed due to COVID-19 (and tips to help you cope).* The Skill Collective. https://theskillcollective.com/blog/coronavirus-new-normal

Crowley, L. (2020, July 8). *Adaptation to The New Normal – Practical Challenges & Tips.* Intuition. https://www.intuition.com/adaptation-to-the-new-normal-practical-challenges-tips/

Czeisler, M. É. (2020). Mental Health, Substance Use, and Suicidal Ideation during the COVID-19 Pandemic. MMWR. *Morbidity and Mortality Weekly Report, 69*(32). https://doi.org/10.15585/mmwr.mm6932a1

Danner, D. D., Snowdon, D. A., & Friesen, W. V. (2001). Positive emotions in early life and longevity: Findings from the nun study. *Journal of Personality and Social Psychology, 80*(5), 804–813. https://doi.org/10.1037/0022-3514.80.5.804

Delpino, F. M., da Silva, C. N., Jerônimo, J. S., Mulling, E. S., da Cunha, L. L., Weymar, M. K., Alt, R., Caputo, E. L., & Feter, N. (2022). Prevalence of anxiety during the COVID-19 pandemic: A systematic review and meta-analysis of over 2 million people. *Journal of Affective Disorders, 318,* 272–282. https://doi.org/10.1016/j.jad.2022.09.003

Effect Of Negative Thinking: Meaning & Causes. (n.d.). Digit Insurance. Retrieved June 18, 2023, from https://www.godigit.com/health-insurance/mental-health/effect-of-negative-thinking

Emanuel, E. J., Osterholm, M., & Gounder, C. R. (2022). A National Strategy for the "New Normal" of Life With COVID. *JAMA, 327*(3). https://doi.org/10.1001/jama.2021.24282

Emmons, R. A., & McCullough, M. E. (2003). Counting blessings versus burdens: An experimental investigation of gratitude and subjective well-being in daily life. *Journal of Personality and Social Psychology, 84*(2), 377–389. https://doi.org/10.1037/0022-3514.84.2.377

Footprints to Recovery Editorial Staff. (2017, September 20). *Core Beliefs: How They Influence You and What to Do About It. Footprints to Recovery* | Drug Rehab & Alcohol Addiction Treatment Centers. https://footprintstorecovery.com/blog/core-beliefs/

Fran. (2021, April 13). *Gratitude and happiness | The importance of being grateful.* FutureLearn. https://www.futurelearn.com/info/blog/gratitude-and-happiness-importance-being-grateful

Good Therapy. (2011). *Emotion–Focused Therapy.* Goodtherapy.org. https://www.goodtherapy.org/learn-about-therapy/types/emotion-focused-therapy

Grinspoon, P. (2022, May 4). *How to recognize and tame your cognitive distortions.* Harvard Health. https://www.health.harvard.edu/blog/how-to-recognize-and-tame-your-cognitive-distortions-202205042738#:

Harvard Health. (2019, March 21). *Benefits of Mindfulness.* HelpGuide.org. https://www.helpguide.org/harvard/benefits-of-mindfulness.htm

Hawkley, L. C. (2013). Negative Thoughts. *Encyclopedia of Behavioral Medicine,* 1305–1306. https://doi.org/10.1007/978-1-4419-1005-9_1563

HealthDay. (2021). *Health Care After COVID: The Rise of Telemedicine. US News & World Report*; U.S. News & World Report. https://www.usnews.com/news/health-news/articles/2021-01-05/health-care-after-covid-the-rise-of-telemedicine

Hirschlag, A., & Juby, B. (2018, December 18). *How to Cope with Anxiety: 13 Simple Tips.* Healthline. https://www.healthline.com/health/mental-health/how-to-cope-with-anxiety#8-long-term-strategies

How to stop negative thoughts. (n.d.). Spiritual Science Research Foundation. Retrieved June 16, 2023, from https://www.spiritualresearchfoundation.org/spiritual-practice/steps-of-spiritual-practice/personality-defect-removal-and-improvement/how-to-stop-negative-thoughts/?

Hughes, A. (2018, July 5). *8 In-the-Moment Techniques to Cultivate Your Mindfulness Pra.* Yogapedia.com. https://www.yogapedia.com/2/8460/meditation/mindfulness/how-to-be-more-mindful

Hung, C.-L., Lin, Y.-L., Chou, C.-M., & Wang, C.-J. (2023). Efficacy of Aromatherapy at Relieving the Work-Related Stress of Nursing Staff from Various Hospital Departments during COVID-19. *Healthcare, 11*(2), 157. https://doi.org/10.3390/healthcare11020157

Jantz, D. G. (2011, July 7). *How Anxiety Fuels Codependency.* The Center • a Place of HOPE. https://www.aplaceofhope.com/how-anxiety-fuels-codependency/

Johnson, C. (n.d.). *Stuck on Negative Thinking.* Care Counseling. Retrieved June 16, 2023, from https://care-clinics.com/stuck-on-negative-thinking/#:

Killian, J. (2020, May 23). *5 Ways to Overcome Codependency - Anxiety Therapist in New Haven.* Arcadian Counseling. https://arcadiancounseling.com/5-ways-to-overcome-codependence/

Lindberg, S. (2020, November 26). *Self-Improvement Goal Setting Tips.* Verywell

Mind. https://www.verywellmind.com/tips-for-goal-setting-self-improvement-4688587

Locke, E. A. (1968). Toward a theory of task motivation and incentives. *Organizational Behavior and Human Performance, 3*(2), 157–189. https://doi.org/10.1016/0030-5073(68)90004-4

Lucidchart. (2018, February 6). *The Ultimate Goal Setting Process: 7 Steps to Creating Better Goals.* Lucidchart. https://www.lucidchart.com/blog/7-steps-to-creating-better-goals

Marteka. (2019, July 15). *12 Ways to Recognise Negative Thoughts.* Benevolent Health. https://benevolenthealth.co.uk/12-ways-to-recognise-negative-thoughts/

Mayo Clinic Staff. (2021, July 29). *Stress relief from laughter? It's no joke.* Mayo Clinic. https://www.mayoclinic.org/healthy-lifestyle/stress-management/in-depth/stress-relief/art-20044456

McEvoy, P. M., Watson, H., Watkins, E. R., & Nathan, P. (2013). The relationship between worry, rumination, and comorbidity: Evidence for repetitive negative thinking as a transdiagnostic construct. *Journal of Affective Disorders, 151*(1), 313–320. https://doi.org/10.1016/j.jad.2013.06.014

Messina, M. (n.d.). *Identifying Core Beliefs: Dr. Messina & Associates: Clinical Psychologists.* Www.drmessina.com. Retrieved June 20, 2023, from https://www.drmessina.com/blog/identifying-core-beliefs

Miles, M. (2022, January 19). *Adjusting to the new normal: What you can expect.* Www.betterup.com. https://www.betterup.com/blog/new-normal

MIND. (2021). *Coronavirus: the consequences for mental health The ongoing impact of the coronavirus pandemic on people with mental health problems across.* In Mind. https://www.mind.org.uk/media/8962/the-consequences-of-coronavirus-for-mental-health-final-report.pdf

Morrison, D. (2023, January 7). *Shifting Your Perspective On Fear.* Medium. https://medium.com/running-relentless/shifting-your-perspective-on-fear-6facfbfaab7c

National Institute of Mental Health. (2021). *Chronic Illness and Mental Health: Recognizing and Treating Depression.* National Institute of Mental Health. https://www.nimh.nih.gov/health/publications/chronic-illness-mental-health

O'Keefe, P. A., Dweck, C. S., & Walton, G. M. (2018). Implicit Theories of Interest: Finding Your Passion or Developing It? *Psychological Science, 29*(10), 1653–1664. https://doi.org/10.1177/0956797618780643

Outreach. (2021, November 19). *Negative Thought Patterns and Depression.* Sage Neuroscience Center. https://sageclinic.org/blog/negative-thoughts-depression/

Panigrahi, S. (2022, April 23). *Develop Optimism and Mental Resilience to Conquer Anxiety.* Www.stanleywellnesscentre.com. https://www.stanleywellnesscentre.com/practitioner-blogs/develop-optimism-and-mental-resilience-to-conquer-anxiety

Parker, S. (2023, April 13). *Anxiety as the Path to Freedom | Psychology Today.* Www.psychologytoday.com. https://www.psychologytoday.com/intl/blog/embracing-unrest/202303/anxiety-as-the-path-to-freedom

Peck, S. (2019, February 12). *Why a Growth Mindset is Essential for Learning - Learn to Code in 30 Days.* https://learn.onemonth.com/why-a-growth-mindset-is-essential-for-learning/

Perlmutter, A. (2020, February 10). *3 Ways to Manage Worry by Perspective Shifting | Psychology Today.* Www.psychologytoday.com. https://www.psychologytoday.com/intl/blog/the-modern-brain/202002/3-ways-manage-worry-perspective-shifting

Phillips, B. D. (2011, February 6). *ATTITUDES, VALUES, AND BELIEFS 态度价值和信仰 - 心理学空间.* Www.psychspace.com. https://www.psychspace.com/psych/viewnews-3772

Pizzagalli, D. A. (2010). Frontocingulate Dysfunction in Depression: Toward Biomarkers of Treatment Response. *Neuropsychopharmacology, 36*(1), 183–206. https://doi.org/10.1038/npp.2010.166

Pohle, A. (2021, March 23). *How to Develop Self-Discipline and Find Motivation.* Wall Street Journal. https://www.wsj.com/articles/how-to-build-self-discipline-and-find-motivation-11610561933

Polemis, J. (n.d.). *Reframing Defeating Beliefs and Language – Coaching for Leadership.* Coaching for Leadership. Retrieved June 20, 2023, from https://wp.nyu.edu/coaching/skills/reframing/

Prem, R., Scheel, T. E., Weigelt, O., Hoffmann, K., & Korunka, C. (2018). Procrastination in Daily Working Life: A Diary Study on Within-Person Processes That Link Work Characteristics to Workplace Procrastination. *Frontiers in Psychology, 9.* https://doi.org/10.3389/fpsyg.2018.01087

Primeau, M. (2021, September 15). *Your powerful, changeable mindset.* Stanford Report. https://news.stanford.edu/report/2021/09/15/mindsets-clearing-lens-life/

Psychology Today. (2017). *Procrastination | Psychology Today*. Psychology Today. https://www.psychologytoday.com/us/basics/procrastination

Richter, F. (2021, February 4). *COVID-19 has caused a huge amount of lost working hours*. World Economic Forum; World Economic Forum. https://www.weforum.org/agenda/2021/02/covid-employment-global-job-loss/

Riopel, L. (2019, June 14). *The Importance, Benefits, and Value of Goal Setting*. PositivePsychology.com. https://positivepsychology.com/benefits-goal-setting/

Romanoff, S. (2022, December 6). *6 Ways to Use Anxiety as a Source for Growth | Psychology Today*. Www.psychologytoday.com. https://www.psychologytoday.com/us/blog/life-in-transition/202212/6-ways-use-anxiety-source-growth

Rousou, K. (2020, June 13). *14 Simple Tips to Form Good Habits and Stay Consistent*. Mindful Wonderer. https://mindfulwonderer.com/how-to-form-good-habits/

Saeed, S. A., Cunningham, K., & Bloch, R. M. (2019). Depression and Anxiety Disorders: Benefits of Exercise, Yoga, and Meditation. *American Family Physician, 99*(10), 620–627. https://www.aafp.org/pubs/afp/issues/2019/0515/p620.html

Sara. (2022, February 8). *Consistency and Creating Habits*. MeVSme. https://mevsme.com.au/consistency/

ScienceDaily. (2020, September 24). *Loneliness levels high during COVID-19 lockdown: More than a quarter of respondents were defined as lonely in UK survey*. ScienceDaily. https://www.sciencedaily.com/releases/2020/09/200924141620.htm

Scott, E. (2019). *How to Make Mindfulness Your Way of Life*. Verywell Mind. https://www.verywellmind.com/mindfulness-exercises-for-everyday-life-3145187

Scott, E. (2022, May 24). *The Toxic Effects of Negative Self-Talk*. Verywell Mind. https://www.verywellmind.com/negative-self-talk-and-how-it-affects-us-4161304

Selva, J. (2018, March 16). *5 Worksheets for Challenging Negative Automatic Thoughts (+PDF)*. PositivePsychology.com. https://positivepsychology.com/challenging-automatic-thoughts-positive-thoughts-worksheets/

Serafini, G., Parmigiani, B., Amerio, A., Aguglia, A., Sher, L., & Amore, M. (2020). The psychological impact of COVID-19 on the mental health in the general population. *QJM, 113*(8), 531–537. https://doi.org/10.1093%2Fqjmed%2Fhcaa201

Serra, R., Borrazzo, C., Vassalini, P., Di Nicolantonio, C., Koukopoulos, A. E., Tosato, C., Cherubini, F., Alessandri, F., Ceccarelli, G., Mastroianni, C. M., D'Ettorre, G., & Tarsitani, L. (2022). Post-Traumatic Stress Disorder Trajectories the Year after COVID-19 Hospitalization. *International Journal of Environmental Research and Public Health, 19*(14), 8452. https://doi.org/10.3390/ijerph19148452

Shah, P. F. (2019, July 7). *21 Empowering Beliefs I Choose To Live My Life By.* Thrive Global. https://community.thriveglobal.com/21-empowering-beliefs-i-choose-to-live-my-life-by/

Shatz, I. (2019). *Why people procrastinate: The psychology and causes of procrastination – Solving Procrastination.* Solvingprocrastination.com. https://solvingprocrastination.com/why-people-procrastinate/

Shonin, E., & Van Gordon, W. (2013). Searching for the Present Moment. *Mindfulness, 5*(1), 105–107. https://doi.org/10.1007/s12671-013-0248-0

Steel, P. (2007). The Nature of procrastination: a meta-analytic and Theoretical Review of Quintessential self-regulatory failure. *Psychological Bulletin, 133*(1), 65–94. https://doi.org/10.1037/0033-2909.133.1.65

Stevens, A. (2022, August 15). *What Effect Does Negative Thinking Have on Health?* Absolute Awakenings Treatment Center. https://absoluteawakenings.com/what-effect-does-negative-thinking-have-on-health/

Stoerkel, E. (2019, February 4). *The Science and Research on Gratitude and Happiness.* PositivePsychology.com. https://positivepsychology.com/gratitude-happiness-research/#science-and-research

Sutton, J. (2017, December 5). *15 Anxiety Worksheets and Workbooks for Teens, Kids, & Adults (PDF).* PositivePsychology.com. https://positivepsychology.com/anxiety-worksheets/

Tallon, M. (2020, April 13). *10 Simple Ways to Practice Mindfulness In Our Daily Life.* Moniquetallon.com. https://moniquetallon.com/10-simple-ways-to-practice-mindfulness-in-our-daily-life/

Tarlac Agricultural University. (2022). *PEH12 Q3 Mod1 Moving On Adapting The New Normal v4-1-1 - Physical Education and Health (H.O.P. 4) - Studocu.* Studocu. https://www.studocu.com/ph/document/tarlac-agricultural-university/bachelr-of-animal-science/peh12-q3-mod1-moving-on-adapting-the-new-normal-v4-1-1/18447499

Team Soulveda. (2023, May 11). *How to Overcome Procrastination with Effective Planning.* Soulveda. https://www.soulveda.com/wellbeing/power-of-planning-overcoming-procrastination-through-organisation/

Temple, J. L., Bernard, C., Lipshultz, S. E., Czachor, J. D., Westphal, J. A., & Mestre, M. A. (2017). The Safety of Ingested Caffeine: A Comprehensive Review. *Frontiers in Psychiatry, 8*(80). https://doi.org/10.3389/fpsyt.2017.00080

THC Editorial Team. (2021, October 14). *Present-Moment Awareness: Overview, Benefits, and Practice.* The Human Condition. https://thehumancondition.com/present-moment-awareness/

Tracy, B. (2022, September 16). *How to Develop Self Discipline to Succeed.* Brian Tracy. https://www.briantracy.com/blog/personal-success/self-discipline/

Utah State University. (2022, February 7). *Growth Mindset: A New Tool to Help with Anxiety and Depression.* Extension.usu.edu. https://extension.usu.edu/mentalhealth/articles/growth-mindset-a-new-tool-to-help-with-anxiety-and-depression

Villines, Z., & Wade, D. (2022, August 23). *Core beliefs: Definition, how to identify, and more.* Www.medicalnewstoday.com. https://www.medicalnewstoday.com/articles/core-beliefs#how-to-identify

Washington, N. (2020, January 31). *7 Tips to Cope with COVID-19 Anxiety.* Psych Central. https://psychcentral.com/anxiety/coronavirus-anxiety-ways-to-cope-with-fear#seeking-help

WebMD Editorial Contributors. (2021, April 9). *What Is Acceptance and Commitment Therapy?* WebMD. https://www.webmd.com/mental-health/what-is-acceptance-and-commitment-therapy

Wellbeing. (2022, March 18). *How has the COVID-19 pandemic affected mental health?* Zurich.com. https://www.zurich.com/en/media/magazine/2021/5-ways-the-covid-19-pandemic-has-impacted-mental-health

World Health Organization. (2020, October 5). *COVID-19 disrupting mental health services in most countries, WHO survey.* World Health Organization. https://www.who.int/news/item/05-10-2020-covid-19-disrupting-mental-health-services-in-most-countries-who-survey

World Health Organization. (2022, March 2). *COVID-19 pandemic triggers 25% increase in prevalence of anxiety and depression worldwide.* World Health Organization. https://www.who.int/news/item/02-03-2022-covid-19-pandemic-triggers-25-increase-in-prevalence-of-anxiety-and-depression-worldwide

Youn, S. J., & Marques, L. (2018, October 23). *Intensive CBT: How fast can I get better?* Harvard Health Blog. https://www.health.harvard.edu/blog/intensive-cbt-how-fast-can-i-get-better-2018102315110

Zou, Y., Li, P., Hofmann, S. G., & Liu, X. (2020). The Mediating Role of Non-reactivity to Mindfulness Training and Cognitive Flexibility: A Randomized Controlled Trial. *Frontiers in Psychology, 11.* https://doi.org/10.3389/fpsyg.2020.01053

www.ingramcontent.com/pod-product-compliance
Lightning Source LLC
Chambersburg PA
CBHW051538020426
42333CB00016B/1986